Professional and Practice-based Learning

Volume 26

Professional and practice-based learning brings together international research on the individual development of professionals and the organisation of professional life and educational experiences. It complements the Springer journal *Vocations and Learning: Studies in vocational and professional education.*

Professional learning, and the practice-based processes that often support it, are the subject of increased interest and attention in the fields of educational, psychological, sociological, and business management research, and also by governments, employer organisations and unions. This professional learning goes beyond, what is often termed professional education, as it includes learning processes and experiences outside of educational institutions in both the initial and ongoing learning for the professional practice. Changes in these workplaces requirements usually manifest themselves in the everyday work tasks, professional development provisions in educational institution decrease in their salience, and learning and development during professional activities increase in their salience.

There are a range of scientific challenges and important focuses within the field of professional learning. These include:

– understanding and making explicit the complex and massive knowledge that is required for professional practice and identifying ways in which this knowledge can best be initially learnt and developed further throughout professional life.
– analytical explications of those processes that support learning at an individual and an organisational level.
– understanding how learning experiences and educational processes might best be aligned or integrated to support professional learning.

The series integrates research from different disciplines: education, sociology, psychology, amongst others. The series is comprehensive in scope as it not only focusses on professional learning of teachers and those in schools, colleges and universities, but all professional development within organisations.

More information about this series at http://www.springer.com/series/8383

Madeleine Abrandt Dahlgren • Hans Rystedt
Li Felländer-Tsai • Sofia Nyström
Editors

Interprofessional Simulation in Health Care

Materiality, Embodiment, Interaction

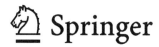 Springer

Editors
Madeleine Abrandt Dahlgren
Department of Medical and Health Sciences
Linköping University
Linköping, Sweden

Li Felländer-Tsai
Department of Clinical Science,
Intervention and Technology (CLINTEC)
Division of Orthopedics and Biotechnology
Karolinska Institutet
Stockholm, Sweden

Hans Rystedt
Department of Education, Communication
and Learning
University of Gothenburg
Gothenburg, Sweden

Sofia Nyström
Department of Behavioural Sciences
and Learning
Linköping University
Linköping, Sweden

ISSN 2210-5549   ISSN 2210-5557   (electronic)
Professional and Practice-based Learning
ISBN 978-3-030-19541-0   ISBN 978-3-030-19542-7   (eBook)
https://doi.org/10.1007/978-3-030-19542-7

This Springer imprint is published by the registered company Springer Nature Switzerland AG.
The registered company address is: Gewerbestrasse 11, 6330 Cham, Switzerland

Series Editors' Foreword

A key goal of this book series is to contribute to discussions about and processes for improving the enactment of occupational capacities through professional practice-based experiences. A related goal is associated with understanding and enhancing the contributions that different kinds of experiences can make to the formation and continuity of those occupational practices. The volumes in this series have contributed a range of perspectives, approaches and outcomes to these discussions. This volume continues that tradition through considerations of how simulation-based activities can contribute to enhancing occupational practices in which working and learning progresses inter- and intra-professionally within healthcare settings. The procedural concern here is to enhance patient safety through improving the quality of collaborative working and learning by healthcare workers. The conceptual concern here is to understand how such working and learning can be understood more fully as a process of interdependence amongst practitioners, and how such co-working and learning progresses, in what ways and for what outcomes. Added here are the ways in which technology comes to mediate and support that process. Perhaps only through such considerations, focused empirical work and detailed analysis will our understanding of human capacities, their enactment and evaluation transcend from either wholly individualised or wholly socialised accounts.

The sections comprising this book are drawn from a large collaborative study hosted by three institutions that have longer and solid traditions of making contributions to understanding the development of professional capacities through interprofessional practices (i.e. Linkoping), dedicated focuses on improving healthcare practices (Karolinska) and the use of technology in working and learning (Gothenburg). These collaborations have been informed and enriched by contributors from other institutions who bring explanatory concepts. The attempt to utilise, accommodate and optimise these different contributions is exercised within the organisation of the sections of the book and chapters within it, highlighted by a process of dual considerations and separate commentaries. Each of these sections provides an overview, statements about procedural matters (e.g. how to conduct inquiries or how to analyse data), proposing and advancing particular explanatory accounts, and also offering perspectives on how educational or work practice might be enhanced. This structuring is particularly helpful as it provides focused considerations of particular phenomena (e.g. team-based approaches to simulation, use of video recordings, doing simulations) through description, analysis and commentary.

In these ways, this volume offers contributions to discussions about the goals for, processes of and outcomes of professional and practice-based learning in a manner that is highly consistent with the ambitions of this book series.

University of Brisbane   Stephen Billett
Brisbane, Australia
University of Regensburg   Hans Gruber
Regensburg, Germany
University of Paderborn   Christian Harteis
Paderborn, Germany

Preface

Interprofessional Simulation in Health Care: Materiality, Embodiment, Interaction

This book is about interprofessional learning in simulation-based education in health care with the intended audience of researchers, university teachers and practitioners interested in simulation pedagogy for the health professions. The contents of the book will provide a research-based problematization of simulation as a pedagogical technology for practice-based learning in health care education and practice. It will do so against the backdrop of the changing views and current discourses on professional learning, and the global call for the need for health care education reform. The call for reform includes interprofessional learning and collaboration as a means of resolving the expected shortage of health care professionals and to ensure patient safety for the future. The book will provide theorizations and empirical examples as a contribution to the debate on what directions simulation pedagogy needs to take to accommodate for such learning objectives.

The Authors of This Book

The book builds on a four-year collaborative research project funded by the Swedish Research Council, Educational Sciences 2013–2016 between successful research environments at Linköping University (LiU), Karolinska Institutet (KI) and the University of Gothenburg (GU). The collaboration provides opportunities to draw on different research expertise, experiences, ideas and perspectives. The research team at Linköping University, Faculty of Health Sciences, have specialized in research on learning in higher/professional education, interprofessional education and the relationship to work life. The research team at the Center for Advanced Medical Simulation and Training (CAMST) at Karolinska Institutet specializes in research in medical simulation, focusing on the development of simulation-based training and on the impact on the development of clinical skills. The research at the University of Gothenburg has been carried out within The University of Gothenburg Learning and Media Technology Studio (LETStudio), a priority area for promoting interdisciplinary research within the learning sciences, that focuses on the relation between new technologies for learning and the development of professional expertise. In addition, external and international experts involved in research on simulation have been involved in the research project at various stages as critical friends, in comparative and joint analyses and as discussants. Hence, the book will provide findings from research conducted in national and international collaboration between interprofessional teams of researchers. The teams comprise health care professionals, professional educators in health programs and educational researchers. The unique collaborative design and focus on praxis-oriented methodologies of this project fills a knowledge gap in the existing research literature and contributes to the enhancement of knowledge on pedagogy in virtual environments and the design and integration of technology-enhanced learning in curricula of professional education in medicine and allied health.

The Structure of the Book

The reader will find that the structure of the book is modelled like a conversation – each chapter is introduced and commented on by different invited international experts and critical friends alike. The chapters often have two different sections, authored by different author teams. The intention is that they be read in sequence, but each section can also be read as a stand-alone contribution on its respective topic. The book also has a methodological ambition to showcase how simulation practices could be researched by the use of practice-oriented theoretical frameworks and video data. Furthermore, the sequence of chapters in the book mirrors dimensions and phases of the simulation practice that our research has identified as important for the planning, execution and follow-up of education and learning with simulation.

Acknowledgements

The editors would like to thank the Swedish Research Council, Educational Sciences, for the funding of the project "Interprofessional Simulation-based Education for the Health Professions" (Dnr 721-2012-5450), which made this research possible. We also would like to thank all participants, students, professionals, instructors, who have willingly participated in the different studies.

Linköping, Sweden	Madeleine Abrandt Dahlgren
Stockholm, Sweden	Li Felländer-Tsai
Linköping, Sweden	Sofia Nyström
Gothenburg, Sweden	Hans Rystedt

Contents

Part I   Setting the Scene

1   **Why This Book?** 3
Madeleine Abrandt Dahlgren, Li Felländer-Tsai, Sofia Nyström,
and Hans Rystedt

2   **Understanding Interprofessional Simulation Practice** 9
Hans Rystedt, Madeleine Abrandt Dahlgren, and Michelle Kelly

3   **Video as a Tool for Researching Simulation Practices**.............. 31
Madeleine Abrandt Dahlgren, Elin Nordenström,
Donna Rooney, and Hans Rystedt

**Part II   The Practices of Interprofessional Simulation – Preparing,
Doing, Observing and Reflecting**

4   **Preparing for Team Work Training in Simulation**................. 59
Michelle Kelly, Sissel Eikeland Husebø, Hans Rystedt,
Cecilia Escher, Johan Creutzfeldt, Lisbet Meurling,
Li Felländer-Tsai, and Håkan Hult

5   **Doing Interprofessional Simulation** 91
Nick Hopwood, Song-ee Ahn, Sanna Rimpiläinen,
Johanna Dahlberg, Sofia Nyström, and Ericka Johnson

6   **Observing Interprofessional Simulation**........................ 115
David Boud, Sofia Nyström, Madeleine Abrandt Dahlgren,
Johanna Dahlberg, Donna Rooney, Michelle Kelly,
and Dara O'Keeffe

7   **Reflecting on Interprofessional Simulation** 139
Sissel Eikeland Husebø, Madeleine Abrandt Dahlgren,
Samuel Edelbring, Elin Nordenström, Torben Nordahl Amorøe,
Hans Rystedt, and Peter Dieckmann

Part III   Simulation Pedagogy Re-Visited

8   **Bodies in Simulation**.   175
   Peter Dieckmann, Ericka Johnson, and Nick Hopwood

9   **Advancing Simulation Pedagogy and Research**.   197
   Hans Rystedt, Madeleine Abrandt Dahlgren,
   Li Felländer-Tsai, and Sofia Nyström

Part I
Setting the Scene

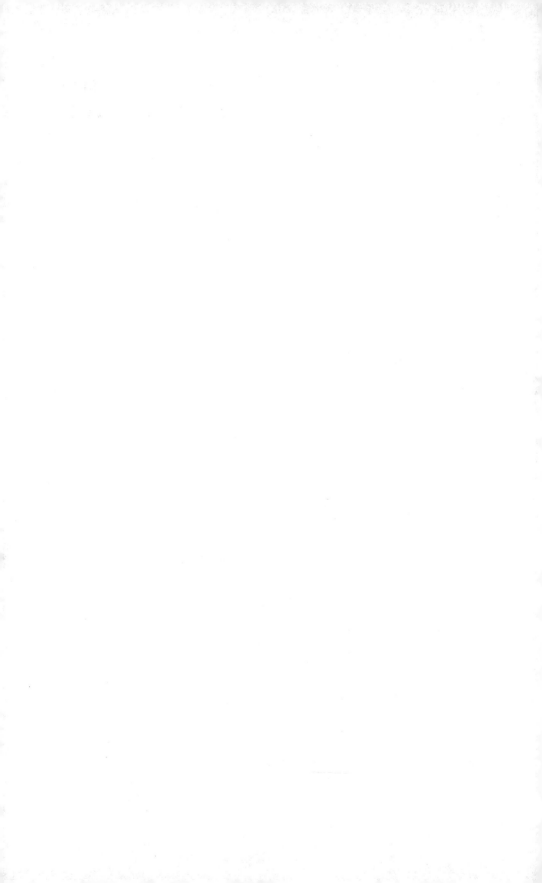

Chapter 1
Why This Book?

Madeleine Abrandt Dahlgren, Li Felländer-Tsai, Sofia Nyström, and Hans Rystedt

1.1 Responding to Change

Our opening chapter raises a question of why a book, entitled "Learning together: Interprofessional learning in simulation in health care" is needed. Seen from a broad outlook, the world of health care practice is changing, comprising several challenges for health professionals. Health care services and professionals around the world are under pressure coping with limited resources, access to health care, and equity problems. At the same time, the demands to improve quality in practice and enhance patient safety are crucial. These conditions present knowledge and learning challenges and have implications for education and continuous development of health professionals. Interprofessional collaboration and teamwork has been emphasized as one of the means, but also challenges in order to accomplish a sustainable and safe health care system, requiring a renewal of professional health care education (Frenk et al. 2010; WHO 2010). The Lancet Commission report (Frenk et al. 2010) lists a number of aspects that affect the conditions for sustainable health care globally. Demographic changes, e.g. the ageing workforce in health care and the increase in people living with chronic deceases combined with advances in medical expertise and healthcare technologies, mean that more people are surviving life-threatening conditions. The need for health care services will increase while the

M. Abrandt Dahlgren (✉) · S. Nyström
Linköping University, Linköping, Sweden
e-mail: madeleine.abrandt.dahlgren@liu.se; sofia.nystrom@liu.se

L. Felländer-Tsai
Karolinska Institutet, Stockholm, Sweden
e-mail: li.tsai@ki.se

H. Rystedt
University of Gothenburg, Gothenburg, Sweden
e-mail: hans.rystedt@ped.gu.se

© Springer Nature Switzerland AG 2019
M. Abrandt Dahlgren et al. (eds.), *Interprofessional Simulation in Health Care*,
Professional and Practice-based Learning 26,
https://doi.org/10.1007/978-3-030-19542-7_1

recruitment of qualified health care professionals is limited. These are some of these challenges that health professionals for the twenty-first century need to be prepared to tackle in their work (Frenk et al. 2010). In addition, the number of injuries induced by mistakes and miscommunication between health professionals, make the improvement patient safety highly prioritized on the agenda for future health care. Several aspects of teamwork have been identified as potential causes to unsuccessful outcome (Manser 2009). In spite of extensive investments and efforts the estimated number of patients harmed does not seem to change (Landrigan et al. 2010).

Following the call for change of health care organization and delivery and the need of health care education reform, the inclusion of interprofessional learning as part of the undergraduate education of all health professions is also emphasized. Professional education in healthcare has been claimed to be organized in "professional silos" (McNair 2005) to the detriment of learning of interprofessional collaborative skills. Interprofessional collaborative skills are hence seen as necessary in health care in order to resolve the expected shortage of health care professionals and to ensure patient safety for the future (Frenk et al. 2010).

1.1.1   Interprofessional Education

Interprofessional education (IPE), in which students learn from, with and about each other, in competency-based curricula has been promoted globally as a necessity to meet the present demands on health care (WHO 2010). Future health professionals need to demonstrate competency in a number of aspects, of which three are (1) to integrate and enact disciplinary knowledge in clinical settings, (2) to understand and respond to practical, intellectual and ethical problems in clinical work, and (3) to collaborate in interprofessional teams. A suggested solution for educational programs in health has been to adopt competency-based curricula responsive to rapidly changing needs, and to exploit the power of information technology for learning (Frenk et al. 2010). This call for change presents a number of challenges for professional health care educators in undergraduate programs and in continuing professional education in the endeavor to foster interprofessional collaboration, and to provide possibility for the training of clinical skills in risky situations without jeopardizing patient safety. Global issues of particular importance for health care educators that the Frenk report (2010) are how to improve patient safety, and how to establish effective teamwork and collaborative practice as part of the solution to this. A further challenge concerns how to establish partnership models of healthcare delivery that take into account the perspective of the health care consumer (Costanza 2015; Frenk et al. 2010; WHO 2013). Simulation-based education has become an important educational tool for teaching and learning such competences.

Interprofessional education (IPE), has been defined as curricular activities in which students from different professional programs learn from, with and about each other (CAIPE 2002; Thistlethwaite 2012) to improve quality of care and services. To accomplish IPE, a close collaboration between health care education and health care services is needed to expand arenas for and to make possible clinical placements where students can learn collaboration and teamwork with patients in practice (Frenk et al. 2010). Interprofessional learning and collaboration as a practice in education and health care is seen as a complex phenomenon that is under-theorized and under-researched (Barr et al. 2005; Cooper et al. 2001; Freeth et al. 2001; Fox and Reeves 2015). In this book, we are focusing on a specific educational arrangement for interprofessional learning, i.e. simulation-based interprofessional simulation with technology enhanced, full-scale manikin scenarios.

Simulation scenarios has become a common means in attempts of overcoming the complex of nested problems in interprofessional learning and collaboration, both in training of professionals as well as in education of students. Simulation has a long tradition in health care education, in the form of physical models for imitating human anatomy or disease to help students learn various discrete skills in medicine and nursing. and has "come of age" as a teaching method in medical education (Norman 2014). The use of simulation spans from the training of discrete skills to the mimicking of complex practices. The ideas of how to arrange simulation for educational purposes of training a practice have migrated into health care from other areas than education. Medical simulation is influenced by military simulation and procedures for safety in aviation, dating back to the early twentieth century (Singh et al. 2013). The migration of simulation into professional health care has brought about a tradition of the pedagogy for a simulation exercise as following a predefined set of stages that has been labelled briefing, simulation and debriefing (e.g. Dieckmann et al. 2009). Simulation of health care work, where a technologically advanced manikin replaces the patient, is increasingly being used in undergraduate programs as a means for dealing with scarce resources, including shortage of clinical practice placements. Simulation hereby has become a complement to clinical placements as well as a way to arrange a safe environment for training of clinical and interprofessional skills for professional practice in health (Cant and Cooper 2010). Against the backdrop of the increasing use of simulation as a means of professional and interprofessional learning, the need to understand how to arrange these activities, in order to best support students' learning, becomes an important research issue. The benefits of using simulations for learning purposes have often been motivated by the possibilities to train the management of potentially dangerous situations under controlled conditions without putting peoples' health at risk. A fundamental assumption is that simulated activities could mirror the complexities involved in clinical work by allowing participants to act and interact in work-like settings. Whilst the debate on the effect of fidelity on learning has been going on for decades, the search for general effects have been downplayed, and has been replaced by notions more adapted to educational purposes. For instance, Hamstra et al. (2014) suggested the notion of "functional task alignment", to put attention to in what ways the design of simulations could meet more specific learning objectives. Still, there is a need for more empirical studies on what such an alignment means in interprofessional simulation-based learning environments.

1.1.2 Interprofessional Simulation

There is a growing body of research supporting the hypothesis that training in simulators can enhance team performance (McGaghie et al. 2010), but previous research provides us with scarce evidence of how such interprofessional collaboration is learned and enacted in simulation practice. Reviews of research on interprofessional simulation-based training show that studies focusing on the practice of simulation in undergraduate programs are still less common (Gough et al. 2012; Palaganas et al. 2014). Instead, research in interprofessional education (IPE) and simulation in undergraduate training have predominantly concerned evaluation of courses, learners' perspective of IPE, and teamwork outcomes (Cook et al. 2011). Some studies also focused on the learners' attitudes and their learning about the roles and skills of other professions or disciplines (Gough et al. 2012).

Most research on the use of simulations for professionals' team training focus on the effects of simulation-based training on performance, whilst the educational intervention itself, the practice of simulation, is largely unexplored. Although it is important to know if simulations are effective educational environments, further knowledge on the practice itself is necessary to open up the black box and answer questions on why simulation training can function as powerful means for improving team communication and performance. The theoretical and empirical starting point of this book is that the unpacking how simulations work in practice can inform both research and education. We see it far from given what the simulation is a simulation of, and how this is related to clinical practices. In this book, we will argue that such fundamental issues are at the core of understanding the conditions for learning in interprofessional simulation practice. This, in turn, necessitates facilitation methods that are sensitive to how facilitators and trainees in collaboration make sense of simulated events and constitute the simulation as a simulation of healthcare practice. Hence, we argue that in order to understand the complexity of interprofessional learning, there is a need for alternative perspectives that allow for relational and contextual descriptions and analyses of practices. There is a need for explorative research on how arrangements for the interprofessional health care practices during interprofessional simulation enable students' learning and collaboration.

1.1.3 The Outline and Content of the Book

In Chap. 2, we outline the arguments and main features of the theoretical frameworks we apply, and that situate research on interprofessional simulation practices in different but related practice-oriented views, that has been applied in empirical research across the collaborating teams. Chapter 3 continues with a methodological description of how video is used as a research tool for the study of interprofessional simulation and provide empirical examples of how video has been utilized as a method of qualitative data collection and approaches to analyses. Chapter 4 starts at the first phase of the simulation scenario. The ways of introducing simulation activities and preparing the participants for the following scenarios are broadly acknowledged as important for the opportunities to learn. In this chapter, we showcase methods for elucidating the significance of how participants are prepared for simulations in simulation-based team training.

Chapter 5 takes us further into the enactment of the simulation scenario and explores how the enactment of interprofessional simulation emerges in fluid relationships between different actors. In simulation-based education, it is common not only to participate in the scenario, but also to observe others simulation scenarios for learning. Chapter 6 looks further into the situated conditions of observers and problematize the material conditions required, and the set-up processes needed for observing practice to be fostered. In Chap. 7, we have entered the debriefing phase post-simulation. Here we elucidate how the use of video recordings from scenarios for enhancing reflection can offer insights in how models for feedback are played out and discuss their implications for learning. In the third section of the book, Chap. 8 provides a theoretical and empirical focus on the body of the simulator as designed and perceived, how it is simulated and interacted with. Chapter 9 provides a reflective summary and discussion of the contributions of the book to simulation pedagogy and research. Pedagogical implications and suggestions for future research are provided.

References

Barr, H., Koppel, I., Reeves, S., Hammick, M., & Freeth, D. (2005). *Effective interprofessional education. Argument, assumption & evidence*. Oxford: Blackwell publishing.

CAIPE (2002). Interprofessional education – a definition. www.caipe.org.uk

Cant, R. P., & Cooper, S. J. (2010). Simulation-based learning in nurse education: Systematic review. *Journal of Advanced Nursing, 66*(1), 3–15.

Cook, D. A., Hatala, R., Brydges, R., Zendejas, B., Szostek, J. H., Wang, A., et al. (2011). Technology-enhanced simulation for health professions education: A systematic review and meta-analysis. *Journal of the American Medical Association, 306*(9), 978–988.

Cooper, H., Carlisle, C., Gibbs, T., & Watkins, C. (2001). Developing an evidence base for interdisciplinary learning: A systematic review. *Journal of Advanced Nursing, 35*, 228–237.

Costanza, M. (2015). Measuring the impact of interprofessional education on collaborative practice and patient outcomes. *Journal of Interprofessional Education and Practice, 1*(2), 34–35.

Dieckmann, P., Molin Friis, S., Lippert, A., & Østergaard, D. (2009). The art and science of debriefing in simulation: Ideal and practice. *Medical Teacher, 31*, e-287–ee294.

Fox, A., & Reeves, S. (2015). Interprofessional collaborative patient-centred care: A critical exploration of two related discourses. *Journal of Interprofessional Care, 29*(2), 113.

Freeth, D., Reeves, S., Goreham, C., Parker, P., Haynes, S., & Pearson, S. (2001). 'Real life' clinical learning on an interprofessional training ward. *Nurse Education Today, 21*(5), 366–372. https://doi.org/10.1054/nedt.2001.0567.

Frenk, J., Chen, L., Bhutta, Z., Cohen, J., Crisp, N., Evans, et al. (2010). Health professionals for a new century: Transforming education to strengthen health systems in an interdependent world. *Lancet, 376*(9756), 1923–1958.

Gough, S., Hellaby, M., Jones, N., & MacKinnon, R. (2012). A review of undergraduate interprofessional simulation-based education. *Collegian, 19*(3), 153–171.

Hamstra, S. J., Brydges, R., Hatala, R., Zendejas, B., & Cook, D. A. (2014). Reconsidering fidelity in simulation-based training. *Academic Medicine, 89*(3), 387–392. https://doi.org/10.1097/ACM.0000000000000130.

Landrigan, C. P., Parry, G. J., Bones, C. B., Hackbarth, A. D., Goldmann, D. A., & Sharek, P. J. (2010). Temporal trends in rates of patient harm resulting from medical care. *New England Journal of Medicine, 363*(22), 2124–2134.

Manser, T. (2009). Teamwork and patient safety in dynamic domains of healthcare: A review of the literature. *Acta Anaesthesiologica Scandinavica, 53*(2), 143–151. https://doi-org.e.bibl.liu.se/10.1111/j.1399-6576.2008.01717.x.

McGaghie, W. C., Issenberg, B. S., Petrusa, E. R., & Scalese, R. J. (2010). A critical review of simulation-based medical education research: 2003–2009. *Medical Education, 44*, 50–63.

McNair, R. (2005). The case for educating healthcare students in professionalism as the core content of interprofessional education. *Medical Education, 39*(5), 456–464.

Norman, G. (2014). Simulation comes of age. *Advances in Health Sciences Education, 19*(2), 143.

Palaganas, J. C., Epps, C., & Reamer, D. (2014). A history of simulation-enhanced interprofessional education. *Journal of Interprofessional Care, 28*(2), 110–115.

Singh, H., Kalani, M., Acosta-Torres, S., El Ahmadieh, T. Y., Loya, J., & Ganju, A. (2013). History of simulation in medicine: From Resusci Annie to the Ann Myers Medical Center. *Neurosurgery, 73*(4), 9–14.

Thistlethwaite, J. (2012). Interprofessional education: A review of context, learning and the research agenda. *Medical Education, 46*(1), 58–70.

World Health Organization. (2010). *Framework for action on interprofessional education and collaborative practice*. Geneva: WHO.

World Health Organization. (2013). *WHO education guidelines 2013. Transforming and scaling up health professionals' education and training*. Geneva: WHO.

Chapter 2
Understanding Interprofessional Simulation Practice

Hans Rystedt, Madeleine Abrandt Dahlgren, and Michelle Kelly

2.1 Introduction

Today the advantages of simulations for developing the skills necessary for effective interprofessional teamwork are broadly acknowledged. However, there is less consensus on what and how participants in interprofessional simulations learn, and there is a lack of theoretical understanding of how learning could be understood and researched. The ultimate question, if interprofessional simulation training could improve clinical practice, has been hard to answer in terms of causal relationships. Instead, much attention has been paid to the effects of interprofessional simulations on attitudes and knowledge (Gough et al. 2012). The results so far indicate that interprofessional simulation is well received and that the outcomes are promising (Dennis et al. 2017). Questions, however, are raised about when the most appropriate time to implement interprofessional learning is, including simulation (Kozmenko et al. 2017). Whilst much effort is devoted to study the effects of the simulation intervention, that is assumed to cause changes, the situation itself is largely dismissed. Consequently, the practice of simulation is "black boxed" which implies a quest for more in-depth knowledge on the process of learning and the conditions necessary for students to develop their knowledge of interprofessional teamwork. The aim of this chapter is to outline the theoretical and methodological foundations

H. Rystedt (✉)
University, of Gothenburg, Gothenburg, Sweden
e-mail: hans.rystedt@ped.gu.se

M. Abrandt Dahlgren
Linköping University, Linköping, Sweden
e-mail: madeleine.abrandt.dahlgren@liu.se

M. Kelly
Curtin University, Perth, Australia
e-mail: michelle.kelly@curtin.edu.au

© Springer Nature Switzerland AG 2019
M. Abrandt Dahlgren et al. (eds.), *Interprofessional Simulation in Health Care*,
Professional and Practice-based Learning 26,
https://doi.org/10.1007/978-3-030-19542-7_2

9

for "opening the black box" of practice and direct the analytical focus to what takes place when people are learning together in and through interprofessional simulations.

Before delving into the traditions underpinning the major methodological approaches suggested in this book, we will revisit some of the major theoretical traditions permeating much research on learning and simulations this far. Our contention is that there is not one answer to what learning is or how it should be researched (Hager and Hodkinson 2009). Neither is there a need for a unified theory. Quite the contrary, we argue for the need for different theories that can give richer knowledge on how we can develop and integrate simulations as approaches to learning. In doing this, it is important to attend to the differences between the basic assumptions on knowledge and learning that the theories rely on and the methods they imply in order to acknowledge their contributions. Following Kuhn, one can argue that there are paradigmatic differences between research traditions with respect to the problems they address, the methods in use, and what constitutes legitimate results (Kuhn 1962). In research on learning, significant incompatibilities can be boiled down to differences in the unit of analysis, for instance if the analysis is directed to individual mental processes or to social interaction (Säljö 2009). On this premise, we will put focus on the unit of analysis in comparing research traditions within simulation and learning, how it is underpinned by basic assumptions on cognition and its methodological implications. In doing this, our ambition is to explicate how the turn to practice, proposed in this book, can contribute to new knowledge on the learning potential of interprofessional simulation that has been largely overlooked in much research this far. With that in mind, some of the major research traditions permeating research on simulation and learning are presented as a basis for outlining what the turn to practice would imply.

Much research on learning has been carried out under an umbrella of theories related to *cognitivism*. This tradition was a reaction to behaviourism, in which observable behavior was treated as the unit of analyses, and learning conceived as a result of new connections between stimulus and response. Whilst this assumption implied a view on learning as a result of external influences, the cognitivist tradition directed interest to inner mental processes, acknowledging the individual mind as the primacy for cognition and learning. This view is related to *constructivism*, premised on the assumption that the human mind actively gives meaning and order to the reality we are engaged in (e.g. Piaget 1970). In short, this means that knowledge is constructed by the individual and that the analytical interest is directed to how people process information to make sense of their experiences. In line with the focus on inner mental processes, theories have emerged that conceptualize our understandings and actions as shaped by the individual's *mental models*, functioning as representations of the surrounding world. Learning, from this point of view involves changes of the persons' existing mental models and cognitive structures (Johnson-Laird 2006). In research on simulation and learning, these traditions have been influential for studies of cognitive processes involved in medical decision-making and problem-solving (e.g. Gaba 2018).

In the wake of cognitivism and constructivism, much research has been carried out with the notion of *transfer* as the common denominator. Broadly speaking, transfer refers to how something learnt in one situation could be transferred to another situation. Much research in this field has been designed as randomized controlled trials (RCT) in which better performance of the experimental group compared to the controls is seen as evidence of learning in terms of transfer (see Hager and Hodkinson 2009). This research tradition has increased our understanding of the impact of simulation training, for instance the impact of training with simulators on performance in more advanced simulators or, in some cases, in clinical settings (e.g. Boet et al. 2014). However, there are many obstacles to overcome in order to find evidence of transfer, for instance to define the intervention, what constitutes relevant outcome variables and to state the causal relationships between them. Although this line of research has provided important empirical contributions, we think it leaves out the process of learning itself and neglects the contextual nature of cognition and learning. For instance, when the analytical perspective is directed to how participants act and interact in simulations, it is evident that what could appear to be the same intervention might include rather dissimilar activities (Linell and Persson Thunqvist 2003), implying that the consequences for learning are rather open-ended. On this background, we argue that there is a need for problematizing the intervention itself and to "open the black box" as pointed out above.

Another influential theoretical contribution to the scholarship of healthcare simulation with a focus on individual mental processes, has been Kolb's theory of *Experiential learning* (Kolb 1984). Learning, from this point of view, takes place through a cyclic process including four discrete phases, in which (1) concrete experiences (e.g. from simulations) provide (2) a basis for reflection, leading to (3) conceptual abstraction and (4) abstract experimentation, which in turn, could (5) imply transformations of new experiences. Whilst this framework has been highly influential for informing adult education and the design of simulation training, it has also been critiqued for being a merely theoretical construction building on concepts from diverse traditions such as pragmatism, psychoanalysis, gestalt psychology and neurophysiology that are both incompatible with each other and inadequately transformed (e.g. Miettinen 2000). However, the widespread influence of the theory puts attention to important issues that need to be empirically substantiated, for instance how participants when performing interprofessional simulations reflect on one's experiences, conceptualize those experiences and how these phases are interconnected.

To sum up, a wide range of methods for research on learning through simulations has provided a substantial body of knowledge on the conditions for learning and its effects. We would argue that many of the core issues, briefly presented above, can be deepened by methods that "open the black box" and put the analytical focus on the practice of interprofessional simulation itself. Further, we have argued that the dominating theoretical approaches so far might be too narrow in their scope to allow for such an endeavor, pointing to the need for additional theoretical approaches. Below we will present such theoretical frameworks, their methodological implications and what kind of answers these approaches could provide.

2.2   Turning to Practice

Practice oriented approaches have in common that knowledge and learning are integral aspects of social practices, including individuals, culture and artefacts. In contrast to cognitivism, knowledge cannot be limited to mental or abstract representations residing in the individual mind that are ready to be applied in any possible situation. Instead, the practice view implies that knowledge is inherent in social situations in which people act, solve everyday problems etc. by means of culturally developed tools and practices. In the context of healthcare, for instance, an ordinary activity, such as making a diagnosis, is not only bound up with medical knowledge, but also with institutional and professional responsibilities, use of information from investigations and procedures, forms of documenting, etc. Not the least, as pointed out by Bowker and Star (1999), our knowledge of the world is mediated by the ways it is categorized, something that is an inherent part of professional knowledge and conduct. It would be almost impossible to imagine how healthcare work could be done without all the medical equipment involved and the terminologies and categories permeating professional and interprofessional communication, documentation and decision-making.

The turn to practice in research on learning has various theoretical roots and here we will mainly deal with two approaches that permeate much of the empirical analyses presented in this book. One of them is emanate from theories on *situated action* and is informed by ethnomethodology (EM) and conversation analysis (CA) (Heath and Luff 2000), whilst the other one is based on *practice theory* (Schatzki 2012). Some fundamental assumptions on learning are shared between the approaches, such as social practices as the unit of analysis and thereby also as the primordial site for analyzing learning. But there are also differences with respect to theoretical foundations and their analytical consequences. The aim here is not to unify theories, but rather acknowledge the range of insights in the practice of interprofessional simulation that a turn to practice could contribute to. From this point of departure, we will outline some basic assumptions on learning in practice underpinning the two approaches, respectively. Next, the similarities and differences between the approaches and their analytical consequences will be summarized.

2.2.1   Learning in Practice from a Situated Perspective on Action

The approach to video-based studies focusing on *situated action* is to a large extent informed by the ground-breaking work of Suchman (1987). Whilst her work on plans and situated actions has revolutionized research on human-machine interaction in fields like workplace studies (Heath et al. 2010) and Computer Supported Collaborative Learning (Stahl 2012), it has also been highly influential in studies of learning and instruction in healthcare settings (e.g. Koschmann 2013).

2.2.1.1 From Mental Processes to Situated Action

In contrast to the prevailing cognitive model of human conduct in psychology and cognitive science, Suchman (1987) argued that human conduct cannot only be understood as a result of inner mental processes. Through analyses of interactions between users and an advanced copy-machine she abandoned the prevailing cognitivist view of human cognition and conduct as the execution of plans residing the individual mind. Instead, Suchman showed how enacting plans, in the form of rules, scripts or mental schemata, depends on the contingencies of the situation. Suchman takes the example of going down a rapid stream by canoe. You can have an overall plan for the route to follow, but to really travel down the stream you also need to account of the innumerable conditions that cannot be anticipated in advance, such as currents, rocks, depth of water etc. Plans, in this sense, can serve as a means for guiding actions, but cannot themselves predict every possible situation for their application. Neither can they stipulate what actions that should follow. This implies that the individual mind as the unit of analysis is replaced by situated action, i.e. interaction with others in the technological surround and the innumerable forms of contingencies involved in practical understanding and conduct. Consequently, the analyst's focus is put on how people orient to these contingencies in the conduct of their actions. In analyzing simulations, it means that the focus is put on how the participants, facilitators and learners alike, orient to one another and to features of the technological surround to understand and go on with the activities they are involved in. Explanations like the participants do something "in order to" achieve something are thus abandoned and replaced by an analytical focus on the details of their actual conduct in the midst of action.

The situated perspective on action proposed in this book draws of a number of assumptions and analytical concerns in ethnomethodology (Garfinkel 1967) and conversation analysis (Sacks 1992). A basic assumption in ethnomethodology is that the origins of social order and intersubjectivity can be found in "orders of ordinary action", i.e. the wide range of various methods people employ in making sense of the activities they are engaged in. From this follows that the researchers should avoid imposing their own theoretical explanations or concepts on data. Although this statement could be interpreted as a rejection of theories, it represents a strong theoretical position that social conduct and order is structured by *members' methods*, i.e. "...the things members routinely do to create and recreate the various recognizable social actions or social practices" (Rawls in Garfinkel 2002, p. 6). Further, these methods are *accountable*, i.e. designed in ways that they are recognizable and intelligible for other members of a community. Furthermore, the members' methods are observable for researchers alike and the primary source for understanding how intersubjectivity and social order are accomplished in situ. This means that the ways in which members of a community accomplish common understanding and social order is already there, available for empirical analyses. As a consequence, ethnomethodology informed analyses avoid imposing preconceived categories like mental models, intentions, social structures, culture, ideology, power and so on to explain human understanding and conduct. Or as expressed by Schegloff (1991, p. 51):

> The point is not that persons are somehow not male or female, upper or lower class, with or without power, professors and/or students. [...] There is still the problem of showing from the details of the talk or other conduct in the materials that we are analyzing that those aspects of the scene are what the parties are oriented to. This does not mean that such aspects do not affect people's thinking and conduct, but they are only subjected to analysis if the participants under scrutiny visibly orient to these aspects.

2.2.1.2   Language and Social Interaction

In the wake of ethnomethodology, the development of conversation analysis has led to an increasing interest of language use and social interaction. Conversation analysis paved the way for rigorous and detailed analyses of how the order of social worlds is constituted, turn by turn, through the sequential organization of talk-in-interaction (Sacks et al. 1974). The sequential organization of talk-in-interaction, how the understanding of a turn or action is displayed by the ways it is responded to in the subsequent turn, provides an intrinsic feature of how people accomplish shared understanding and joint actions. This implies that the meaning of an utterance or action cannot be understood in isolation but needs to account for how the sequential order of utterances provides a context for participants to understand the situation at hand and, most important, how every next turn is potentially context renewing. Put in a simulation context, this analytical focus can highlight how the meaning of an on-going simulation can be changed in every next turn and how the participants' understandings of the activity will have a direct impact on how it is played out. An example on how the meanings of simulations can shift in moment-to-moment interactions can be illustrated by a study of the training of professional trauma teams (Rystedt and Sjöblom 2012). The results point to how the simulation is regularly upheld as a work-related activity by keeping to ordinary work routines and treating the manikin as a representation of a real patient. For instance, a question by the acting physician to the other team-members in the simulation "has he been on trauma CT?" can initiate an orientation to the simulation as work related. But such a question can also expose a discrepancy between the conditions of the simulation and the ordinary work routines in which the physician is expected to know the results of the CT. Therefore, when another team member, in response to the prior turn, asks "haven't you been there", the dissimilarities with work routines are topicalized. Such glitches, in turn, can imply breakdowns in which the activity shifts from a work related one to a focus on the conditions of the simulation itself. The point here is that such transformations of the activity can take place in moment-to-moment interactions and that simulations, as other activities, can take new directions in every next turn. Linell and Persson Thunqvist (2003) argue that these transformations instantiate how participants can move in and out of different framings of simulations, which accentuates their open-ended and ambiguous character. Thereby, analyses of the sequential organization of talk-in-interaction could provide additional empirical contributions to discussions on the significance of "suspension of disbelief" and fiction/reality cues in simulation (Dieckmann 2007).

2.2.1.3 Embodied Actions and Artefacts

In addition to talk, the sequential organization of action and interaction also involves visual conduct, gestures and the interaction between people and artefacts such as tools and technologies in the environment (Goodwin 1994; Heath and Luff 2000). As stated above, various forms of medical equipment routinely feature in healthcare work, decision-making and coordination between staff members. In a study of anesthetic teams Hindmarsh and Pilninck (2002, p. 139) point toward "the critical importance of analyzing embodied conduct, not just language or talk, when examining co-present organizational activities". When inducing anesthesia, the team members have to coordinate a series of tasks, often in sequence but also partly overlapping. Such an alignment of conduct demands both the performance of individual tasks and to make their actions "visible and available to their colleagues" (p. 148). The conduct and coordination of such actions is enabled by an orientation to the onset of an action as projecting a certain set of other actions to follow, for instance administering an injection of anesthetic and slipping a mask onto the patient's face in a timely manner to increase the oxygen level in the blood before intubation. In terms of Hindmarsh and Pilnick (2002), the performance of actions functions as collaborative resources for the coordination of the activity. Most importantly, much of this coordination is conducted tacitly, pointing to the indexicality of actions, gestures and talk to project specific meaning, intelligible for the other members of the team. This, in turn, shows how competent teamwork relies on the members' abilities, not only to perform individual actions, but also to notice, read, anticipate and act on each other's actions. Therefore, the development of the competencies necessary for teamwork involves a sensitivity to the talk and bodily conduct of others in the domain.

The analytical focus on the alignment of talk, gestures and embodied action in the coordination of teamwork has also been applied in research on learning in simulation-based environments. In a study of resuscitation training of nursing students most actions were found to be accomplished through simultaneous talk and embodied actions, such as body torque, pointing, taking positions etc. (Eikland Husebø et al. 2011). Similarly, as pointed out by Hindmarsh and Pilnick (2002), talk directed to the patient/manikin functioned as a shared resource for the team by projecting what was going on, and what actions should follow. In stating that the "patient" was unconscious and to prepare for the onset of CPR the students seldom explicitly asked each other what should be done. Instead, the lack of response from the manekin provided a shared sign for the team members to take action and prepare for CPR. Through concerted actions, like flattening the bed, removing the pillows and placing the patient in a supine position, they displayed to each other both the existence of cardiac arrest and what actions should follow. Therefore, the analytical attention to details of the participants' on-going and emergent interactions could reveal much of the seen but unnoticed features involved in learning the competencies needed for proficient teamwork. Often the focus in educating for the health professions is put on correctly following given algorithms. An important argument in this book is that many of the critical but often unnoticed features of teamwork seldom are highlighted in research on simulation-based learning. In parallel to Suchman (1987), skillful performance does not only rely on executing plans, like algorithms for CPR, but to acknowledge the innumerable contingencies involved in upholding "the tacit order of teamwork". In addition, we would argue, that simulation provides both a site for analyzing the significance of talk-in-interaction and embodied conduct in instruction, and to explore its potential for learners to become competent participants in interprofessional teams. As exemplified in this book, the alignment of talk and embodied conduct is a central feature of instruction in briefings, both in demonstrating how tasks should be performed and to elaborate on the similarities and dissimilarities between the simulator and human patients (see Sect. 4.2 this volume). Further, Sect. 4.3 (this volume) showcases how gestures and actions are essential in-scenario instructions and provide decisive resources for the participants' understanding of the scenarios and how to proceed in line with the intended learning objectives.

2.2.1.4 Professional Vision

The significance of analyzing talk and embodied conduct is further addressed in a series of studies on *professional vision*. The notion of professional vision, as used here, was originally elaborated in a series of anthropological studies on expert witnesses, archeologists, and marine scientists (Goodwin 1994, 1995, 2018). These studies bring attention to the ways in which professions are able to interpret what they see in congruent ways through practices of coding and highlighting. By applying such practices, they are building and contesting professional vision, consisting of "socially organized ways of seeing and understanding events that are answerable to the distinctive interests of a particular social group" (Goodwin 1994, p. 606). From this view follows that the analytical interest is directed to how professionals in healthcare observe, identify and categorize the concrete signs of patients in specific situations, such as in surgery (Koschmann et al. 2011), radiology (Alaç 2008; Slack et al. 2007) and anesthesiology (Sanchez Svensson 2007). Regularly it involves the appropriate use of instruments and interpretations of the data they provide. This point can be illustrated by an empirical example from a study in which pairs of nursing students used a desktop simulation in their training to become nurse anesthetists (Rystedt and Sjöblom 2012). In this case, the task involved how to maintain physiological equilibrium and balance effects and side-effects of anesthetics. When an unacceptable fast heart rate was observed during anesthesia, displayed by an icon on the screen, this was recurrently interpreted as a sign of pain. To confirm such interpretations, the students also checked icons displaying depth of anesthesia, delivery of anesthetic gases and blood-pressure before adding additional anesthetics (which could have solved the problem). This specific interpretation can be seen as the application of a particular practice of coding in anesthesia practice in which a patient's health status is assessed via the monitors and gauges in the operating room where typical patterns of signs are highlighted and identified as significant. Or as Rawls (in Garfinkel 2002, p. 166) puts it: "Things' are made to appear as objects of a sort only when oriented toward in specifiable ways in the context of a practice.". In sum, this implies that competent performance in a situation involves the application of professional practices for seeing and interpreting events as meaningful in relation the task at hand.

The notion of professional vision is also relevant for understanding the conditions necessary for participants to learn from observing simulations. When novices are observing others' activities in simulation scenarios, or in retrospect through video recordings, it is often far from evident for them what is relevant from a professional point of view. A strong argument for using video in post-simulation debriefing is that the participants would see how they performed instead of relying on how they thought they performed (Fanning and Gaba 2007). This could be the case, but as shown by a series of empirical studies, such viewing, especially for novice learners, necessitates guided instructions to interpret the events in congruent ways that are relevant to the learning objectives of the activity (see Erickson 2007). As demonstrated in a study of Johansson et al. (2017), a close analysis of the interaction between facilitators and students in video-assisted debriefings shows how the students' interpretations of what was shown on video clips were shaped by a wide range of contingencies, such as the facilitators' questions, the students' interactions and the video itself (see also Sect. 7.3 this volume). The facilitators opening question after showing a video clip, implied that the answers were to be found in what just was shown. In doing this, events in the scenarios were not only re-actualized, but also re-assessed and re-contextualized. These transformations of what the video actually showed were to a large extent enabled by contrasting the students' appearances on the video with their immediate experiences after the scenario. From a methodological point of view, the close analysis of questions and answers and the ways in which these were linked to the video clips, enabled an understanding of how facilitators and students were able to see the same thing and link this to professionally relevant aspects of teamwork. In all, it unpacks, on a detailed level, the all over importance of systematic feedback and how debriefings could be designed to benefit from video use.

2.2.2 Learning in Practice Through a Practice Theory Lens

Hager et al. (2012) argue that discourses of the nature of professional knowledge and learning at large are changing. The dominating scientific, technical rationalities of professional practice as simply the application of theoretical knowledge, possessed by individuals, are being challenged. Many attempts are made to re-organize and re-think educational design in order to prepare students better for professional health care practice and to reduce the "theory-practice gap". Introducing a practice theory perspective of pedagogy on simulation in professional health care education and practice might allow a new gaze on a field that for a long time been has been dominated by cognitive discourses about how to improve students' learning in higher education. In this section, we discuss the study of professional and practice-based learning from a sociomaterial, practice theory perspective. Such perspectives are increasingly being used in order to understand professional practice and learning in new ways (Fenwick et al. 2011; Fenwick and Abrandt Dahlgren 2015) and have also been the theoretical framing and basis for several of the studies cited in this book.

Practice theories constitute a family of theories that, although they stem from different traditions, share some common features. Nicolini (2009, p. 1394) summarizes these similarities as a joined belief in that:

- Practices constitute the horizon within which all discursive and material actions are made possible and acquire meaning; that practices are inherently contingent, materially mediated, and that practice cannot be understood without reference to a specific place, time, and concrete historical context (Engeström 2000; Latour 2005; Schatzki 2002, 2005).
- While practices depend on reflexive human carriers to be accomplished and perpetuated, human agential capability always results from taking part in one or more sociomaterial practices (Reckwitz 2002).
- Practices are mutually connected and constitute a nexus, texture, field, or network (Giddens 1984; Schatzki 2002, 2005; Latour 2005; Czarniawska 2007). Social co-existence is in this sense rooted in the field of practice, both established by it and establishing it. At the same time, practices and their association perform different and unequal social and material positions, so that to study practice is also the study of power in the making (Ortner 1984).

2.2.2.1 A Practice Theory Perspective and Focus

Adopting a practice theory perspective directs our focus to, in Schatzki's words (2002), how the nexus of actions in practice hang together and are integrated. Schatzki also suggests that practices are relational and bundled with material entities and arrangements (Schatzki 2012). Our attention and analyses aim at revealing how these practice-arrangement bundles facilitate and organize the structure and content of learning in different ways. Hopwood et al. (2014) argue that such a view implies an understanding of a curriculum as sociomaterial. This means that the curriculum is being enacted, rather than conceived as the execution of a priori defined statements in course outlines and learning objectives. The view of practices as relational means that practices are shaped relationally through how we act and interact both socially and through how these actions and interactions are bundled with the physical environment in a strong sense. Material arrangements and set-ups are not seen just as passive structural features or a passive container for the actions. On the contrary, materials and things are seen as dynamic and integrated with human activities in ways that also act on practice. An illustrative example from our studies of interprofessional simulation with students was when an electrical plug in the simulation control room had been mistakenly pulled out. The interprofessional team of students working around the manikin suddenly noticed that the vital signs on the computer monitor had gone blank, and immediately changed their practice into a resuscitation effort (Nyström et al. 2016a). The outcome of the research with a practice theory approach will portray how the role of things, bodily actions and learning are tightly intertwined as the practice unfolds.

2.2.2.2 Attention to Bodies in Professional Practice

Kinsella (2015) has suggested that a focus on the role of the body in professional practices, in simulated or naturalistic settings, might enable educators and learners to draw attention to other dimensions of knowledge and interactions, that are not easily accessible through cognitive perspectives, "...dimensions that might help us illuminate, understand and investigate other types of knowledge that are relevant to everyday practices" (p. 294). Recognising the role of the body in knowledge production in practice goes beyond a focus on the individual practitioner, in the clarification of how the performance of a practice is constituted by the relational nature of material arrangements and professional bodies (Kinsella 2015). The findings from Hopwood et al. (2016) illustrate how the patient's body is enacted in manikin-based interprofessional simulation practice.

> What is interesting pedagogically in simulation is not what the manikin or other technologies can do or how realistic they are, but how they are made intelligible in practices that bring about learning. Our account is one of multiple bodies being simulated—through doings and sayings bound together with materiality (p. 170).

Frequently, human sized manikins are used in simulations to represent patients, particularly useful when the intent of scenarios is to incorporate medical procedures such as insertion of tubes, or to perform CPR and to defibrillate. The highest technical simulators offer a range of human like features including reactional physiological features, programmed or real time vocal responses (via a participant or faculty member) and so on. The complexities of the "body in the bed" afford a multiplicity of meanings throughout the simulation as Hopwood et al. (2016) and Nyström et al. (2016a) describe. To start, the manikin can be viewed as a technical body as the lifelike capabilities are made known to participants during the briefing, morphing into a clinical body as an additional layer – a persona – is introduced, that being the patient's name, medical and social history, and so on. Nyström et al. (2016a) also describe this as the manikin turning into a medical body, as the students' actions and interactions in relation to the manikin had a strong focus on the medical condition (see also Sect. 5.3). As the simulation unfolded, Hopwood et al. (2016) noticed the emergence of a human body as participants provided therapeutic touch and engaged in conversations about levels of pain or comfort. Similar findings were reported in Nyström's et al. study (2016a). The clinical body re-emerged when procedures were required in the ebb and flow of the scenario, and the technical body presented again, when physiological responses to treatment were measured. These multiple forms of the manikin, and the varying interplay of participants with one or more particular body forms, shines perspective on how the material aspects of simulations can afford opportunities for learners to experience a spectrum of clinical practices in a more holistic rather than piecemeal approach.

2.2.2.3 Practices and Arrangements Co-constitute Each Other

Practices would not exist without the material entities and arrangements they deal with, nor would most material entities and arrangements exist without these practices. The physical environment is thereby more than a group of things or a context or setting for activity. Instead, practices and arrangements co-constitute each other. Such a perspective can help us understand how and why particular activities are more or less likely to happen as the manifold of actions unfold (Schatzki 2002). Schatzki uses the term prefiguration to illustrate that the relation between the material and social arrangements will show how the practice is carried out and the materials are being used.

This means that certain sets of activities will become practically intelligible (Schatzki 2012), that is they become functional and useful through the practice with which they are bundled. A lecture room where chairs and tables are organized in horizontal rows and the teachers positioned on a podium can tell us something about what is practically intelligible as we participate in teaching and learning and how this practice will unfold. Such an arrangement will make it easier as a student to sit and silently listen to a lecture, than to discuss in small break-out groups with each other. The arrangement will also make it easier for a lecturer to show a slide-show than to facilitate a focused discussion. A location for debriefing of simulation equipped with comfortable swivel chairs around small coffee tables can make it practically intelligible to have a collegial conversation and a lecture room configuration can make it practically intelligible to invite participants to individual reflections in writing as part of a pre-structured scheme of debriefing (Nyström et al. 2016b). This is not to say that the physical environment always will be bundled with the practices in a causal way, that a certain arrangement will always lead to a particular practice. The causality can work in both ways. People can react to material arrangements in the way we just described, but human actions can always also create, change or re-arrange material entities for their purposes (Hopwood et al. 2014). In other words, arrangements prefigure, i.e. they shape and are shaped by, the emerging practice (Schatzki 2012).

2.2.2.4 Attention to How Activities Are Organized

The research interest in how the nexus of actions in practice hangs together draws our attention to how the practice's activities are organized. Schatzki (2012) suggests that practices are organized through rules, practical understandings, teleo-affective structures and general understandings. These concepts provide directions for our analyses of how the practice-arrangement bundles are linked together in the nexus of actions. In the following, we will give some examples to illustrate how these concepts apply to our analyses. According to Schatzki, actions within a practice are guided by rules that are shared and that regulate the practice. These rules are explicit, formulated directives. Rules are a ubiquitous part of human life, Schatzki argues, they are everywhere and are being constantly produced by humans (2012), even so in professional practice. One example of how rules are bundled with and act on the simulation practice is the ABCDE protocol, that regulates what procedure to follow, actions to be taken and in what order in, for example, a critical trauma scenario. The participants in the interprofessional simulation exercises we have studied explicitly refer to these rules by relating their doings to the protocol as they enact the practice. This means speaking out loud what is being done and a report of the result, e.g. "I am doing A, airways are clear" or "We are on C, circulation is OK". Depending on how the result of the examination according to the protocol turns out, the practice unfolds in different ways. Another example of how rules act on simulation practices is if the debriefing model in use normatively corrects or alters what is being enacted in the debriefing. A debriefing model might normatively state that a debriefing session should start with a reaction phase where participants could defuse emotions (e.g. Rudolph et al. 2006), and the way the model is bundled with the facilitator's actions will change how the practice unfolds in accordance with the model (see Sect. 7.2 for a further elaboration on this issue), in ways that are more or less supporting interprofessional learning in a productive way.

Practical understanding is what is expressed in the enactment of practice, the doings and sayings that constitute how the work is practically carried out. The performances of practices are also relational to the historical and various social contexts in which they evolve, and practical understandings of the same kind of practice might differ between different locations and traditions. One example of how the practical understanding may act on the simulation practice is Johnson's (2007) study of the practice of gynecological examination of the pelvis. A simulator that was developed in the US for medical students and doctors to practice gynecological examination of the pelvis did not function well in a Swedish gynecological practice – the practitioners had different practical understandings of how such an examination should be carried out. The way the simulator was constructed did not allow for the Swedish doctors to perform the examination in accordance with their locally and historically situated practical understandings.

The ways the actions within a practice are carried out are not only guided by practical and general understandings, but also by *teleo-affective structures*. Teleo-affective structures are what makes sense to do, what is acceptable as a professional and ethical conduct. The teleological part of the teleo-affective structure comprises the acceptable means to reach an acceptable end, when carrying on a practice. The affective part of the teleo-affective structure comprises the emotions and moods that people carrying out on a practice should or may acceptably express. One example of how teleo-affective structures emerge in simulation practice is illustrated by what we previously described in this chapter referring to Hopwood et al. (2016) who noticed that participants provided therapeutic touch and talked to the manikin about levels of pain or comfort. A similar finding previously mentioned in the chapter from Nyström et al. (2016a), was when the nursing students tucked the blanket around the manikin's feet as in order to keep them warm. Finally, the nexus of actions is linked to the general understanding of the practice, the purpose of the practice and the ways of working. If we return to our example of the different practical understandings of gynecological examination practice, Johnson (2007) showed that although the general understanding of the purposes of such an examination might be shared across locations, also the construction of a simulator is situated in local and practical understandings.

2.2.2.5   What Will a Practice Theory Perspective Make Visible?

A practice theory perspective makes visible these practices as encompassing a particular pedagogical intention to change how the participants react to the material world, their bodily repertoire of actions, and general understanding of the practice they are participating in. These conceptualizations of professional learning share the ethnomethodological focus of the situated and emergent nature of practice. An important difference is how the role of this theoretical standpoint is played out in the ways the research is conducted. As was outlined in the previous section, in ethno-methodology, the members' methods are used to avoid imposing the researcher's theoretical categories on the empirical data. From a practice theory perspective, the theory instead provides analytical categories that are used for zooming in on certain features of practice (Nicolini 2009) and for zooming out to a broader theoretical understanding in the interpretation of the findings. This can be described as a process of iteration between inductive and theory-driven analyses (Srivastava and Hopwood 2009). Nicolini (2009) describes how the shifting of theoretical lenses through zooming in on aspects of practices can help with articulating e.g. the sayings and doings, the active role of material elements and infrastructure, local methods and micro strategies of concerted accomplishment, or body choreographies. Shifting lenses in zooming out can help to follow the broader practice through trailing connections, e.g. articulate the associations or links between practices, the mediators, the patterns of associations and interests, the local and trans-local effects and the effects of the global on the local (Nicolini 2009, p. 1412).

To summarize, sociomaterial practice theory perspectives suggest alternative views of knowledge as being embodied and relational, intertwined with ethical reasoning and materiality (Gherardi 2009; Green and Hopwood 2015; Kemmis 2009; Schatzki 2002, 2012). In Schatzki's (2002) terms, a practice is an organized nexus of action, a set of bodily doings and sayings. These bodily doings and sayings are organized by a practical understanding of the knowing in a practice. The practical understanding and performance of practice is influenced by rules and, what Schatzki's labels, teleoaffective structures. Rules are explicit normative enjoinings that regulate the actions, while the teleoaffective structures guide the activities in the practice towards a range of acceptable actions and acceptable ends. Furthermore, the performance is influenced by a general understanding, referring to a broader understanding of practice as a whole. It is important to emphasize that the focus in a sociomaterial, practice theory perspective is not on singular things or technologies, but on relationships between human action and material arrangements, and how these relationships emerge and change one another in a practice (Hager et al. 2012; Fenwick and Abrandt Dahlgren 2015; Abrandt Dahlgren et al. 2016). Such a focus has significant implications for how we understand interprofessional simulation-based education. We focus on what these relationships produce in terms of specific actions, habitual practices and learning. While specific relationships might be planned for or anticipated, they are only ever established in a particular course of action. It thus makes sense to regard simulation as an emergent phenomenon, a result of fluid relationships between the social and material as they play out in specific contexts, the outcomes of which may be unpredictable, and at times hard to detect (Abrandt Dahlgren et al. 2016).

2.3 Similarities and Differences Between the Two Approaches

The two approaches have in common an interest in *materiality*, referring to a focus on the ways interaction and learning are bound up with artefacts, objects and other constituents of the material surroundings. Analytically, this implies a focus on the ways in which people interact with the material environment and how artefacts are intertwined with how people communicate, make sense of and act before, during and after simulated scenarios. Since the meaning of simulations cannot be determined in advance but depend on how the interaction between the participants in the material surround unfolds, analyses intend to capture the dynamics of learning and uncover how social and material aspects are intertwined and enter in the processes of joint sense-making. This theoretical stance has rather far-reaching consequences for how the conditions for learning and simulation are conceptualized and understood.

Whilst much prior research in the field of simulation relies on the assumption that the similarities between simulation and the clinical context, in terms of *fidelity*, allows for transfer of knowledge, the turn to practice implies another view. For instance, the writings from Rooney et al. (2015) from a practice theory perspective and others (e.g. Tun et al. 2015; Schoenherr and Hamstra 2017; Hamstra et al. 2014) challenge the current assumptions and meaning of the term 'fidelity'. Beyond the descriptions of the 'grades' (high, medium or low) and breadth of fidelity (environmental, technical, psychological), we highlight the fluid notion of fidelity in that "...[it] is not accomplished in the technology, nor in the pedagogic design, but is an emergent phenomenon that must be constantly worked at, socially and materially, in order to be produced and maintained." (Rooney et al. 2015, p. 8). This means, for instance, that a low technical simulation can elicit a high level of emotional fidelity (Orr et al. 2013) and how simple techniques can boost the level of fidelity in simulations (Nestel et al. 2018; Stokes-Parish et al. 2017). In comparison, from a situated perspective on action, the level of fidelity is to be seen as a result of the participants interactions with each other and the material environment. As, pointed out above, the attention to the sequential organization of interaction can reveal how participants can move in and out of frames, implying quite different stances to the relevance of the simulation for clinical work. These assumptions call for turning to practice and how connections to the clinical setting are constituted by trainees and facilitators in moment-to-moment interactions. Further, video studies of interaction have shown how in-scenario instructions are necessary for trainees to understand scenarios as relevant representations of clinical tasks (Escher et al. 2017), but also how differences between the simulation and the work task could provide resources for instruction and reflection on and about professional practice (Hindmarsh et al. 2014).

The fluid and emergent characteristics of simulations and the level of fidelity challenge many of the prevailing assumptions on *transfer* as a result of similarities between simulations and the targeted work tasks. A major problem with the traditional approach to transfer is that interventions like simulations that at a first glance seem to be the same could be quite different and imply different learning objectives. This implies that the "same" simulations could have quite different outcomes and, thereby, contribute to shed light on the well-known difficulties in defining the outcome measures from simulations (Brydges et al. 2015; McGaghie et al. 2011). Instead of investigating causal relationship between intervention and outcomes, practice-oriented theories imply a focus on simulation as a practice in its own right. The relevance of simulations for the work setting is, from this point of view, not conceptualized as an issue of transfer, but rather how facilitators and participants themselves draw on and re-constitute healthcare practice in and through simulations (see also Johnson 2007).

Further, both approaches acknowledge embodiment as a fundamental aspect of learning and accord it a central analytical place. First, by the way the achievement of joint understanding and coordinated actions involves embodied aspects such as the access to each other's actions, gestures, gazes, body positions and so on. Secondly, by the way simulations offer opportunities for participants to embody experiences of being in situations in which practical actions and cognitive aspects, such as in joint decision-makings, are intertwined. For these reasons, the distinction between "technical skills" and "non-technical skills" is hard to uphold from a practice perspective (see also Gjeraa et al. 2016; Nestel et al. 2011).

Both approaches imply an analytical interest for briefing and "scene setting" and how to match the level of information needed as participants proceed through the scenario, but to also keep the momentum going, and so reach the "desired end point" through adapting instructions to the participants' prerequisites and the situation at hand (Kelly and Guinea 2018). Of specific interest are the "in the moment" decisions in relation to how the simulation is unfolding and in what ways participant actions are in line with the intent of the scenario (see Sect. 4.3). Further, such an analytical interest may involve cultural differences amongst the participants as well as faculty (Kelly et al. in press), and how subtle differences in discourses may affect the learning trajectory (Pitkäjärvi et al. 2012).

But there are also significant *differences* between the two approaches. Whilst both build on strong theoretical positions, the role of theory and the analytical commitments that follow differ. On the one hand, the perspective proposed in the spirit of situated action assume that the constitution of social order is to be found in peoples' ordinary actions and their own methods for dealing with everyday problems. Often, this is connected to detailed analyses of talk-in-interaction and how joint understandings develop turn-by-turn. In studies informed by conversation analysis and ethnomethodology, such analyses are key for unravelling the members' methods for achieving shared understandings and how these are built up sequentially in moment-to-moment interactions. As expressed by Francis and Hester (2004, p. 29) EM/CA analyses seek to "show that members' phenomena and members' methods are available in the talk somehow, and to then make that availability inspectable by the reader" (Francis and Hester 2004, p. 31). In this way, the details of persons' talk and actions upon which the analyses are based can be made available to readers by providing extracts from the data which provide possibilities for the reader to check the validity of the analysis.

On the other hand, from a practice theory perspective, theoretical concepts and their relations plays a prominent role in the analysis, as they provide analytical foci and a frame of reference for the interpretation of how the practice hangs together. A perspective on practice as embedded in and relational to social and material arrangements means that the research interest is directed towards how practices unfold and are enacted – the research interest is also relational – what emerges as practical, intelligible ways of acting and interacting, and what is prefigured through the material set up and social arrangements. The level of analysis is the sayings, doings, relatings and their interconnectedness with the material set-up. Typically, the analysis iterates between empirical observations and theoretical interpretation. The outcome of the research will portray how the role of things, bodily actions such as sayings and doings are tightly intertwined as the practice unfolds. Like in EM/CA analyses, the details from the unfolding practice can be made available to readers by providing empirical material. These details will often comprise of field notes, based on the observations made.

2.4   Conclusions

The ambition with this book is to open up "the black box", to unravel many taken for granted assumptions on learning and show how interprofessional simulation practices are shaped in and through practice. The turn to practice proposed in this chapter relies on a set of analytical commitments:

- The conditions for learning can be understood by analyzing real-time social interaction
- Simulations are emergent in the sense that they develop as a result of the relations between facilitators, participants and the material environment
- Embodiment is a central feature of learning, both with respect to how participants understand the relation between material entities such as simulators and human bodies, and how their understanding develops as a result of embodied actions such as gestures, gazes, positioning etc.

References

Abrandt Dahlgren, M., Hopwood, N., & Fenwick, T. (2016). Theorising simulation in higher education: Difficulty for learners as an emergent phenomenon. *Teaching in Higher Education, 21*(6), 613–627. https://doi.org/10.1080/13562517.2016.1183620.

Alaç, M. (2008). Working with brain scans: Digital images and gestural interaction in fMRI laboratory. *Social Studies of Science, 38*(4), 483–508.

Boet, S., Bould, M. D., Fung, L., Qosa, H., Perrier, L., Tavares, W., et al. (2014). Transfer of learning and patient outcome in simulated crisis resource management: A systematic review. *Canadian Journal of Anesthesia, 61*(6), 571–582.

Bowker, G. C., & Star, S. L. (1999). *Sorting things out: Classification and its consequences.* Cambridge, MA: MIT Press.

Brydges, R., Hatala, R., Zendejas, B., Erwin, P. J., & Cook, D. A. (2015). Linking simulation-based educational assessments and patient-related outcomes: A systematic review and meta-analysis. *Academic Medicine, 90*(2), 246–256. https://doi.org/10.1097/ACM.0000000000000549.

Czarniawska, B. (2007). *Shadowing: And other techniques for doing fieldwork in modern societies.* Copenhagen: Liber and Copenhagen Business School Press.

Dennis, D., Furness, A., Duggan, R., & Critchett, S. (2017). An interprofessional simulation-based learning activity for nursing and physiotherapy students. *Clinical Simulation in Nursing, 13*(10), 501–510.

Dieckmann, P. (2007). Deepening the theoretical foundations of patient simulation as social practice. *Simulation in Healthcare, 2*, 183–193.

Eikland Husebø, S., Rystedt, H., & Friberg, F. (2011). Educating for teamwork – Nursing students' coordination methods in simulated cardiac arrest situations. *Journal of Advanced Nursing., 67*(10), 2239–2255.

Engeström, Y. (2000). Activity theory as a framework for analyzing and redesigning work. *Ergonomics, 43*(7), 960–974.

Erickson, F. (2007). Ways of seeing video: Towards a phenomenology of viewing minimally edited footage. In R. Goldman, R. Pea, S. Barron, & S. Derry (Eds.), *Video research in the learning sciences* (pp. 145–155). Mahwah: Lawrence Erlbaum Associate Publishers.

Escher, C., Rystedt, H., Creutzfeldt, J., Meurling, L., Nyström, S., Dahlberg, J., et al. (2017). Method matters: Impact of in-scenario instruction on simulation-based team training. *Advances in Simulation, 2*(25). doi:https://doi.org/10.1186/s41077-017-0059-9.

Fanning, R. M., & Gaba, D. M. (2007). The role of debriefing in simulation-based learning. *Simulation in Healthcare, 2*(2), 115–125.

Fenwick, T., & Abrandt Dahlgren, M. (2015). Towards socio-material approaches in simulation-based education: Lessons from complexity theory. *Medical Education, 49*(4), 359–367. https://doi.org/10.1111/medu.12638.

Fenwick, T., Edwards, R., & Sawchuk, P. (2011). *Emerging approaches to educational research. Tracing the material*. Abigdon: Routledge.

Francis, D. J., & Hester, S. (2004). *An invitation to ethnomethodology: Language, society and interaction*. London: Sage Publications.

Gaba, D. (2018). Human error in dynamic medical domains. In M. S. Bogner (Ed.), *Human error in medicine* (pp. 197–224). Hillsdale: Lawrence Erlbaum Associates.

Garfinkel, H. (1967). *Studies in ethnomethodology*. Englewoods Cliffs: Prentice Hall.

Garfinkel, H. (2002). *Ethnomethodology's program: Working out Durkeim's aphorism*. Lanham: Rowman & Littlefield Publishers.

Gherardi, S. (2009). *Organisational knowledge: The texture of workplace learning*. Oxford: Blackwell publishing.

Giddens, A. (1984). *The constitution of society*. Berkley: University of California Press.

Gjeraa, K., Jepsen, R. M., Rewers, M., Ostergaard, D., & Dieckmann, P. (2016). Exploring the relationship between anaesthesiologists' non-technical and technical skills. *Acta Anaesthesiology Scandinavia, 60*(1), 36–47. https://doi.org/10.1111/aas.12598.

Goodwin, C. (1994). Professional vision. *American Anthropologist, 96*(3), 606–633.

Goodwin, C. (1995). Seeing in depth. *Social Studies of Science, 25*(2), 237–274.

Goodwin, C. (2018). *Learning in doing: Social, cognitive and computational perspectives*. Cambridge: Cambridge University Press.

Gough, S., Hellaby, M., Jones, N., & MacKinnon, R. A. (2012). A review of undergraduate interprofessional simulation-based education (ipse). *Collegian, 19*(3), 153–170.

Green, B., & Hopwood, N. (Eds.). (2015). *The body in professional practice, learning and education*. Dordrecht: Springer.

Hager, P., & Hodkinson, P. (2009). Moving beyond the metaphor of transfer of learning. *British Educational Research Journal, 35*(4), 619–638.

Hager, P., Lee, A., & Reich, A. (Eds.). (2012). *Practice, learning and change: Practice-theory perspectives on professional learning*. Dordrecht: Springer.

Hamstra, S. J., Brydges, R., Hatala, R., Zendejas, B., & Cook, D. A. (2014). Reconsidering fidelity in simulation-based training. *Academic Medicine, 89*(3), 387–392. https://doi.org/10.1097/ACM.0000000000000130.

Heath, C., & Luff, P. (2000). *Technology in action*. London: Cambridge University Press.

Heath, C., Hindmarsh, J., & Luff, P. (2010). *Video in qualitative research*. London: SAGE Publications Ltd.

Hindmarsh, J., & Pilnick, A. (2002). The tacit order of teamwork: Collaboration and embodied conduct in anesthesia. *The Sociological Quarterly, 43*(2), 139–164. https://doi.org/10.1111/j.1533-8525.2002.tb00044.x.

Hindmarsh, J., Hyland, L., & Banerjee, A. (2014). Work to make simulation work: 'Realism', instructional correction and the body in training. *Discourse Studies, 16*(2), 247–269. https://doi.org/10.1177/1461445613514670.

Hopwood, N., Abrandt Dahlgren, M., & Siwe, K. (2014). Developing professional responsibility in medicine: A sociomaterial curriculum. In T. Fenwick & M. Nerland (Eds.), *Reconceptualising professional learning* (pp. 171–183). London: Routledge.

Hopwood, N., Rooney, D., Boud, D., & Kelly, M. A. (2016). Simulation in higher education: A sociomaterial view. *Educational Philosophy and Theory, 48*(2), 165–178. https://doi.org/10.1080/00131857.2014.971403.

Johansson, E., Lindwall, O., & Rystedt, H. (2017). Experiences, appearances, and interprofessional training: The instructional use of video in post-simulation debriefings. *International Journal of Computer Supported Collaborative Learning, 12*(1), 91–112.

Johnson, E. (2007). Surgical simulators and simulated surgeons: Reconstituting medical practice and practitioners in simulations. *Social Studies of Science, 37*(4), 585–608.

Johnson-Laird, P. (2006). Mental models in cognitive science. *Cognitive Science, 4*(1), 71–115.

Kelly, M., & Guinea, S. (2018). Facilitating healthcare simulations. In D. Nestel, M. Kelly, B. Jolly, & M. Watson (Eds.), *Healthcare simulation education: Evidence, theory and practice* (pp. 143–151). West Sussex: Wiley.

Kelly, M., Ashokka, B., & Krishnasamy, N. (in press). *Cultural conciderations in simulation-based education.*

Kemmis, S. (2009). Understanding professional practice: A synoptic framework. In B. Green (Ed.), *Understanding and researching professional practice* (pp. 19–38). Rotterdam: Sense Publishers.

Kinsella, E. A. (2015). Embodied knowledge: Toward a corporeal turn in professional practice, research and education. In B. Green & N. Hopwood (Eds.), *The body in professional practice, learning and education: Body/practice* (pp. 245–260). Cham: Springer International Publishing.

Kolb, D. A. (1984). *Experiential learning: Experience as the source of learning and development.* Englewood Cliffs: Prentice Hall.

Koschmann, T. (2013). Conversation analysis and collaborative learning. In C. E. Hmelo-Silver, C. Chinn, C. K. K. Chan, & A. O'Donnell (Eds.), *The international handbook of collaborative learning* (pp. 149–167). New York: Routledge.

Koschmann, T., LeBaron, C., Goodwin, C., & Feltovich, P. (2011). 'Can you see the cystic artery yet?' A simple matter of trust. *Journal of Pragmatics, 43*(2), 521–541.

Kozmenko, V., Johnson Bye, E., Simanton, E., Lindemann, J., & Schellpfeffer, S. E. (2017). The optimal time to institute interprofessional education in the medical school curriculum. *Medical Science Educator, 27*, 259–266.

Kuhn, T. S. (1962). *The structure of scientific revolutions* (1st ed.). Chicago: University of Chicago Press.

Latour, B. (2005). *Reassembling the social.* Oxford: Oxford University Press.

Linell, P., & Persson Thunqvist, D. (2003). Moving in and out of framings: Activity contexts in talks with young unemployed people within a training project. *Journal of Pragmatics, 35*(3), 409–434.

McGaghie, W., Draycott, T., Dunn, W., Lopez, C., & Stefanidis, D. (2011). Evaluating the impact of simulation on translational patient outcomes. *Simulation in Healthcare, 6*(7), 42–47. https://doi.org/10.1097/SIH.0b013e318222fde9.

Miettinen, R. (2000). The concept of experiential learning and John Dewey's reflective thought and action. *International Journal of Lifelong Education, 19*(1), 54–72.

Nestel, D., Walker, K., Simon, R., Aggarwal, R., & Andreatta, P. (2011). Nontechnical skills: An inaccurate and unhelpful descriptor? *Simulation in Healthcare, 6*(1), 2–3. https://doi.org/10.1097/SIH.0b013e3182069587.

Nestel, D., Krogh, K., & Kolbe, M. (2018). Exploring realism in healthcare simulations. In D. Nestel, M. Kelly, B. Jolly, & M. Watson (Eds.), *Healthcare simulation education: Evidence, theory and practice* (pp. 23–28). West Sussex: Wiley.

Nicolini, D. (2009). Zooming in and out: Studying practices by switching theoretical lenses and trailing connections. *Organization Studies, 30*(12), 1391–1418. https://doi.org/10.1177/0170840609349875.

Nyström, S., Dahlberg, J., Hult, H., & Abrandt Dahlgren, M. (2016a). Enacting simulation: A sociomaterial perspective on students' interprofessional collaboration. *Journal of Interprofessional Care, 30*(4), 441–447.

Nyström, S., Dahlberg, J., Edelbring, S., Hult, H., & Abrandt Dahlgren, M. (2016b). Debriefing practices in interprofessional simulation with students: A sociomaterial perspective. *BMC Medical Education, 16*(148), 1–8.

Orr, F., Kellehear, K., Armari, E., Pearson, A., & Holmers, D. (2013). The distress of voice-hearing: The use of simulation for awareness, understanding and communication skill development in undergraduate nursing education. *Nurse Education in Practice, 13*(6), 529–535. https://doi. org/10.1016/j.nepr.2013.03.023.

Ortner, S. (1984). Theory in anthropology since the 60s. *Comparative Studies in Society and History, 26*(1), 126–166.

Piaget, J. (1970). Piaget's theory. In P. H. Mussen (Ed.), *Manual of child psychology* (pp. 703–732). London: Wiley.

Pitkäjärvi, M., Eriksson, E., & Pitkälä, K. (2012). The diversity issue revisited: International students in clinical environment. *ISRN Nursing, 2012*, 294138. https://doi.org/10.5402/2012/294138.

Reckwitz, A. (2002). Toward a theory of social practices: A development in culturalist theorizing. *European Journal of Social Theory, 5*(2), 243–263.

Rooney, D., Hopwood, N., Boud, D., & Kelly, M. (2015). The role of simulation in pedagogies of higher education for the health professions: Through a practice-based lens. *Vocations and Learning, 8*(3), 269–285. https://doi.org/10.1007/s12186-015-9138-z.

Rudolph, J., Simon, R., Dufresne, R., & Raemer, D. (2006). There's no such thing as "non- judgemental" debriefing: A theory and method for debriefing with good judgements. *Simulation in Healthcare, 1*(1), 49–55.

Rystedt, H., & Sjöblom, B. (2012). Realism, authenticity, and learning in healthcare simulations: Rules of relevance and irrelevance as interactive achievements. *Instructional Science, 40*(4), 785–798.

Sacks, H. (1992). *Lectures on conversation, volumes I and II.* Edited by G. Jefferson with Introduction by E. A. Schegloff. Oxford: Blackwell.

Sacks, H., Schegloff, E. A., & Jefferson, G. (1974). A simplest systematics for the organization of turn-taking for conversation. *Language, 60*(54), 696–735.

Säljö, R. (2009). Learning, theories of learning and units of analysis in research. *Educational Psychology, 33*(3), 202–208.

Sanchez Svensson, M. (2007). Monitoring practice and alarm technology in anesthesiology. *Health Informatics Journal, 13*(1), 9–21.

Schatzki, T. R. (2002). *The site of the social: A philosophical account of the constitution of social life and change.* University Park: Pennsylvania State University Press.

Schatzki, T. R. (2005). The sites of organizations. *Organization Studies, 26*, 465–484.

Schatzki, T. R. (2012). A primer on practices. In J. Higgs, R. Barnett, S. Billett, M. Hutchings, & F. Trede (Eds.), *Practice-based education: Perspectives and strategies* (pp. 13–26). Rotterdam: Sense.

Schegloff, E. A. (1991). Conversation analysis and socially shared cognition. In L. Resnick, J. Levine, & S. Teasley (Eds.), *Perspectives on socially shared cognition* (pp. 150–171). Washington, DC: American Psychological Association.

Schoenherr, J. R., & Hamstra, S. J. (2017). Beyond fidelity: Deconstructing the seductive simplicity of fidelity in simulator-based education in the health care professions. *Simulation in Healthcare, 12*(2), 117–123. https://doi.org/10.1097/sih.0000000000000226.

Slack, R., Hartswood, M., Procter, R., & Rouncefield, M. (2007). Culture of reading: On professional vision and the lived work of mammography. In S. Hester & D. Francis (Eds.), *Orders of ordinary action* (pp. 175–193). Hampshire: Ashgate.

Srivastava, P., & Hopwood, N. (2009). A practical iterative framework for qualitative data analysis. *International Journal of Qualitative Methods, 8*(1), 76–84.

Stahl, G. (2012). Ethnomethodologically informed. *International Journal of Computer-Supported Collaborative Learning, 7*(1), 1–10.

Stokes-Parish, J. B., Duvivier, R., & Jolly, B. (2017). Does appearance matter? Current issues and formulation of a research agenda for moulage in simulation. *Simulation in Healthcare, 12*(1), 47–50. https://doi.org/10.1097/SIH.0000000000000211.

Suchman, L. (1987). *Plans and situated actions: The problem of human-machine communication.* Cambridge: Cambridge University Press.

Tun, J. K., Alinier, G., Tang, J., & Kneebone, R. L. (2015). Redefining simulation fidelity for healthcare education. *Simulation & Gaming, 46*(2), 159–174. https://doi.org/10.1177/1046878115576103.

Chapter 3
Video as a Tool for Researching Simulation Practices

Madeleine Abrandt Dahlgren, Elin Nordenström, Donna Rooney, and Hans Rystedt

3.1 Introduction

Madeleine Abrandt Dahlgren
Linköping University
Linköping, Sweden
e-mail: madeleine.abrandt.dahlgren@liu.se

This chapter describes various ways of applying and analyzing video as a tool for the study of interprofessional simulation. For our purposes, we will problematize two different projects where video has been utilized as a means of qualitative data collection and analysis. We draw on two empirical research projects, of which the first one is the SIMIPL project, a collaborative project between Linköping University, Gothenburg University and Karolinska Institutet in Sweden. The innovative design of the project, with three research teams, working with the same set of video-recorded simulation sessions from three different sites has allowed us to apply different theoretical frameworks to guide our research questions and analyses. The second research project drawn on is carried out at University of Technology (UTS) in Sydney, Australia. The similarities between the research projects reported on in

M. Abrandt Dahlgren
Linköping University, Linköping, Sweden
e-mail: madeleine.abrandt.dahlgren@liu.se

E. Nordenström (✉) · H. Rystedt
University of Gothenburg, Gothenburg, Sweden
e-mail: elin.nordenstrom@ped.gu.se; hans.rystedt@ped.gu.se

D. Rooney
University of Technology, Sydney, Australia
e-mail: donna.rooney@uts.edu.au

© Springer Nature Switzerland AG 2019
M. Abrandt Dahlgren et al. (eds.), *Interprofessional Simulation in Health Care*,
Professional and Practice-based Learning 26,
https://doi.org/10.1007/978-3-030-19542-7_3

this chapter are that they have been focusing on interprofessional learning and collaboration in simulation-based education with undergraduate students in professional health care programs. Both projects also apply practice-oriented perspectives on simulation. There is also an interconnectedness between the members of two research teams to the extent that some of them have acted as critical friends and as visiting scholars to the respective research groups in Linköping and in Sydney.

The practice-oriented perspective directs the analytical attention towards relationships between human actors, such as bodies, and non-human actors, such as the arrangements of patients' and students' bodies, clinical environments, and protocols in use. The quest for access to details in the participants' verbal and embodied interactions in the material surround calls for video recording as the major method for data collection. The advantage of video recording is that that it provides a sustainable data corpus that can be analyzed from different theoretical interests and perspectives. This body of data can be shared with others and be subjected to collaborative analyses in which preliminary findings could be tried out, contested and refined. As pointed out by Heath et al. (2010, p. 6), video data offer:

> ...opportunities for 'time out', to play back in order to re-frame, re- focus and re-evaluate the analytic case... they allow for multiple takes on the data – to explore issues on different occasions, or to consider the same issue from multiple standpoints.

The capture of people's talk, gestures, conduct and use of material objects provide data that open for analyses that are highly sensitive to the practical conditions of simulations and how participants, in interaction, construe simulations and make sense of the events they are involved in. Further, it allows for analyses that are sensitive to the different actors' perspectives and how these are brought to bear in a situation which necessitates collaborative sensemaking, something that is highly relevant for interprofessional learning. Our theoretical perspectives did thus have implications for the development of the analytical process and the concepts used.

In this chapter, we will highlight the practical, ethical and sustainability considerations necessary when applying video recordings of practices as a research method. In the first section, we describe the careful design and piloting of the methods for collecting video data in order to make up a common pool of empirical data. The pool of data was to be shared between, and subject to different kinds of analyses between the three research partners in the SIMIPL project. In the second subsection, the different modes of doing collaborative analyses of video data in the SIMIPL project and the UTS project two are described and discussed.

3.2 Collecting and Sharing Video Data

Elin Nordenström
University of Gothenburg
Gothenburg, Sweden
e-mail: elin.nordenstrom@ped.gu.se

This section gives a detailed description of considerations related to the use of video data in research, and provides some practical guidelines based on how the SIMIPL project was organized and conducted in this respect. The use of video is motivated by the opportunities to understand the intricate details of how interprofessional simulations are constituted and shaped in practice. This necessitates methods that capture the unfolding interactions between the participants and the technological environment. The rationale is that access to the participants' talk, gestures and practical actions enables studies that are highly sensitive to the practical conditions of simulations and how the different actors' perspectives are played out when performing interprofessional simulation (see Chap. 2). Each of the three research teams participating in the SIMIPL project created a data corpus comprising video recordings of simulation-based training carried out at simulation centers at the research teams' home sites. The own data corpuses provided the main basis for the research teams' analyses, but in addition a common pool of data comprising ten video recordings from each site was created. The data pool served to expand the data material and enabled for comparative studies and contrasting analyses. To ensure that all video data was of equivalent character and sufficient quality, a pilot study aimed at developing a common method for collection and sharing of video data was conducted prior to the start of the SIMIPL project. The pilot study was carried out by one of the research teams whose members had extensive experience of recording and working with video data. In the following, we will describe the how the study was designed, concluding with how the common method and approach to video recording was implemented at the three sites.

3.2.1 Developing a Common Method for Data Collection

In order to develop common methods for collecting, storing and sharing data, a pilot study was conducted the year before the start of the research project by one of the three collaborating research teams. Belonging to an educational research environment with a long tradition of undertaking video-based research, the members of this team had solid experience and collegial support for the development of a common method for collecting and sharing video data. The methodological approach used aligned with the approach of an emerging field of qualitative video-based research concerned with how educational and workplace activities in a range of settings are interactionally organized and practically accomplished (e.g. Koschmann et al. 2011;

Lindwall et al. 2014; Mondada 2003; Rystedt et al. 2011; Rystedt and Sjöblom 2012; Sanchez Svensson et al. 2009). Typically, these studies are based on "naturalistic data", that is:

> ...data collected when the people studied act, behave and go about their business as they would if there were no social scientists observing or taping them. Knoblauch et al. (2006, p. 11)

In total, ten simulation training occasions with different groups of learners conducted during a period of approximately 8 months were video recorded as part of the pilot study. All phases of data collection were conducted, such as application for ethical approval, composing of information about the study to be presented to management at the research site and prospective informants, planning and testing of recording arrangements and equipment, and post-processing and analysis of recorded materials. An iterative workflow was applied, which meant that after each recording occasion some procedures were evaluated and improved. When data collection was completed, the experiences of the pilot study were summarized which resulted in a set of guidelines for the implementation of data collection in the major project. In the following paragraphs, the different phases are described in more detail and the implications for the research project are highlighted.

3.2.1.1 Preparing for Data Collection

Like all data collection, the collection of video data requires a lot of preparation, both in terms of legal, ethical and practical issues. A report on good research practice by the Swedish Research Council (Vetenskapsrådet 2017[1]) listing several legal and ethical matters for video-based research served as a useful guidance for the preparation of data collection. In addition, the literature on video-based interaction research (see Chap. 2) provided a valuable background. The following paragraphs describe some important steps that need to be undertaken prior to data collection.

3.2.1.2 Ensuring Ethical Integrity

Worldwide, there are research ethical codex and laws that researchers are required to follow when undertaking research involving human subjects. Research integrity issues are of particular importance when using video as a tool for research. There is a need for increased awareness of both possibilities and risks regarding digitalization, server ownership and data access. Data storage on servers requires caution regarding third party servers. National and international laws and regulations (e.g. General Data Protection Regulation, GDPR and laws of research ethics) are under constant subject to change and must be considered in order to secure compliance.

---

[1] An earlier version of the report was used as reference by the time the pilot study was planned.

To protect individuals and ensure respect for human dignity in research, Sweden, like many other countries, has a law[2] stipulating that certain research on human subjects must undergo ethical review (Heath et al. 2010; Vetenskapsrådet 2017). This law does not cover all forms of research, however, but only research that involves retrieval and handling of sensitive personal data or is likely to cause physical or psychological impact or in other ways harm the subjects, is required to undergo ethical review. All forms of video recording of individuals involve retrieval of personal data since the recordings can be linked to and enable identification of the recorded individuals. Not all personal data are of sensitive character, however, but only such data that gives information on the subjects' race, ethnic origin, political opinion, religious conviction and the like (Vetenskapsrådet 2017).

The video recordings collected in the pilot study, and later in the research project, comprised health care students and professionals conducting simulation-based training in groups, which was not considered to involve personal data of sensitive character. The Swedish regional ethical review board handling the application for ethical approval therefore decided to approve the study.[3] In addition to meet the law on ethical review, research projects handling any form of personal data are required to follow several national, and possibly also international, rules concerning processing of such data.[4] It is beyond the scope of this section to provide a detailed account of such rules, and readers who intend to undertake research involving processing of personal data are recommended to instead retrieve additional information from national public data protection authorities or equivalent.

3.2.1.3 Establishing Contacts and Coordinating with the Setting Under Study

To gain access to an intended research setting, a first step is to arrange a meeting with the persons responsible for the setting in order to give a brief presentation of the project. In addition to explain project ideas and reasons for undertaking the research, it can be valuable to highlight how the research may benefit the setting, as most parties are more willing to participate in research if they can see it is likely to bring more than an additional workload (Heath et al. 2010, p. 15). As a result of the pilot study, it was considered as important to establish contacts with the management at the simulation centers at an early stage to get their permission to undertake the studies. The researchers and the simulation centers had shared interests in developing favorable conditions for supporting interprofessional learning in simulation-based training, which provided a good basis for collaboration at all three sites. In addition,

---

[2] The Swedish Ethical Review Act (SFS 2003:460) is available in Swedish on http://riksdagen.se/sv/dokument-lagar/dokument/svensk-forfattningssamling/lag-2003460-om-%20etikprovning-av-forskning-som_sfs-2003-460

[3] In Sweden, only research covered by the ethical review act may undergo ethical review.

[4] In EU, processing of personal data is governed by the EU General Data Protection Regulation (https://gdpr-info.eu)

since the simulation centers were located at university hospitals where research was an essential part of the practice, both management and staff had great confidence in the importance of research to develop and improve the practices.

Permission from the management is a prerequisite for the research to progress, but it shall be remembered that permission must also be obtained from the individuals that are to be video recorded. A common assumption is that it is difficult to get permission to video record individuals, but as maintained by Heath et al. (2010) it is typically the research interests rather than the methods that are crucial for this matter. Video-based research concerned with individuals' "…knowledge, reasoning and procedures on which they rely to accomplish their activities…" (Heath et al. 2010, p. 17) is rarely considered as problematic. A focus on uncovering mistakes, errors and failings of individuals, on the other hand, might for obvious reasons be met with greater resistance. Consequently, proper information about the aims and interests of a research study, as well as what participation involves, can be crucial for whether requested individuals approve or deny participation. To provide a background for how the principles employed in the research project were developed, the next paragraph describes how the pilot study was presented to prospective informants.

3.2.1.4 Information Sheet and Consent Form

As stated by the Swedish Research Council (Vetenskapsrådet 2017) information to informants about video-based research should clearly describe the purpose of the research, why video recording has been chosen in front of other forms of data collection, what aspects of the video recordings the researchers intend to analyze, and that participation in the research is voluntary. Since video recording of human subjects involves retrieval of personal data, the name of the data protection officer at the organization responsible for undertaking the research shall also be stated. Furthermore, informants shall be told whether the recordings will be edited in order to anonymize faces and/or voices, if copies will be made of the recordings, and if so, how many, if the recordings will be used for purposes other than research (e.g. for educational purposes), that possible connections between the video recordings and other personal data will be encoded, how and where the recordings will be stored, and for how long they will be kept. Preferably, this information should be provided in both oral and written form and followed by retrieval of the informants' consent to participate in the research, preferably in writing. By giving their written consent, informants certify that they have been informed about what participation in the research involves, and that they may at any time withdraw their consent for the researchers to display, analyze or in other ways use the video recordings.

As part of the pilot study, an information sheet addressing the issues listed above was prepared. For retrieval of written consent for participation in the pilot study, and later in the research project,[5] the form included a separate counterfoil with lines for

---

[5] The hope was that the recordings from the pilot study should be of sufficient quality to be used in the major study, and the approval therefore included participation in both projects.

name, signature and date. In addition to describe aims, interests and methods of the research, and clarify that legal and ethical issues had been properly met, the information sheet aimed to make clear that individuals participating in the study would not run the risk of being shown in bad lights due to a focus on individual achievements. It was thus emphasized that the overall interest of the project was in interprofessional learning in simulation-based training environments, and that analyses of the video recordings would focus on the informants' joint rather than individual performance. The information sheet was sent out in advance to the contact persons of the groups asked to participate in the study, along with a request for them to forward the information to the participants of the groups. The aim was to offer them the opportunity to read through the information in advance, and without the influence of the researchers decide if they wanted to participate in the study. Time for provision of oral and written information about the project and retrieval of written consents was also allocated prior to the start of the simulation training. In consultation with the management at the simulation centers, it was decided that training participants who did not wish to be video recorded should, if possible,[6] be placed in one and the same group that was not video recorded.

3.2.1.5   Recording Arrangements and Equipment

To facilitate the planning of practical arrangements for recording, the research teams undertook visits to the simulation centers prior to their first recording occasions. During these visits, the researchers went through the training facilities together with instructors familiar with the routines and procedures for the simulation training. The purpose was to get an idea of what recording equipment would be needed, and where it could be placed during recording of the simulation training. Finding working positions for cameras and microphones can be a bit of a challenge, especially in small spaces. Positioning, focus, and the number of cameras and microphones used to record the activities will all have impact on the character of the collected data, and thereby also on what kind of analyses can be performed (Heath et al. 2010). In addition, for video recordings to be of high quality there are several issues that need to be taken into consideration, such as camera viewpoint, lighting conditions, and location of sound sources. At the same time, consideration must be given to the activities being recorded, so that the recording equipment or the persons handling it do not disrupt these activities (Heath et al. 2010).

At all three simulation centers, the simulation exercises comprised three parts – briefing, scenario, and debriefing – and were carried out in two different rooms with only short breaks in between. When space is limited, as was the case with these training rooms, the video camera/s must often be placed close to the recorded object/s which might result in a view too narrow to capture everything that is going on. If it is clearly defined what specific details are of interest to the research, record-

---

[6] At some training occasions there was only one group. If someone in the group did not want to be video recorded the video recording was cancelled.

ing of certain features of an activity might be enough (Derry et al. 2010). For the main project, however, the aim was to generate a material that would be useful for researchers with different analytical interests and allow for exploration of a wide range of issues, which required recording of the simulation activities in their entirety. It was anticipated that a dual set of recording equipment would be needed to capture all steps of the simulation sessions, each including one to two video cameras and one or more external microphones.

The rooms where the scenarios were carried out were designed as authentic hospital ward rooms and equipped with standard medical supplies and devices. The patients were represented by full-scale computerized manikin. To capture the simulation exercises it was decided to use one to two cameras placed in fixed positions and using single viewpoints which would not require a camera person remaining nearby the camera/s during recording. In addition to enabling supplementary fieldwork to be undertaken alongside the recording (Heath et al. 2010), leaving the cameras unattended was a prerequisite for the scenarios to be recorded since the simulation centers had established routines of allowing only training participants to be present in the simulation room during scenarios.

The rooms where the debriefings were carried out were rather small, and largely occupied by a tables and chairs. To capture the debriefing activities, we planned to use one or two video cameras, preferably with wide-angle lenses, and external wireless microphones. The cameras would be placed so that they captured both facilitators and training participants, and in case video clips were shown for feedback purposes also the video screen. To obtain good lighting conditions, the recording teams were careful not to direct the cameras against strong light sources, such as windows, since that is likely to result in poor image quality. For all cameras, floor tripods that could be adjusted for height were used. A camera on tripod is likely to give a more stable image than a handheld camera, and it does not require a cameraperson holding the camera throughout the recording session. Moreover, a high tripod reduces the risk that the camera sight is blocked by people moving right in front of the camera.

The quality of the sound might be central to the usability of the video recordings – an analysis of the informants' collaborative activities requires that it is possible to hear what they say when talking to each other. Most video cameras have built-in microphones, but typically these do not provide audio of satisfactory quality. Partly, this is due to the rather poor quality of such microphones, but also to that the video camera tends to be located too far away from the audio source to enable sufficient audio uptake. For this reason, we decided to use external microphones placed as close as possible to the audio sources. There are various types of microphones designed for different purposes, some optimal for recording sound coming from one direction (directional microphones) and others for picking up sound from multiple directions (omnidirectional microphones). When choosing a microphone, it is thus important to consider the direction and character of the sound.

To make sure that the handling of the recording equipment would run smoothly when it was time for recording, the equipment was carefully tested prior to recording. Even persons with extensive experience of handling recording equipment can benefit from double checking how essential features work, such as how to start and stop recording, and how to adjust audio settings, image sharpness, zooming and the like. It can also be useful to test how to fold up tripods and mount cameras, plug in microphones, pull power cables etcetera, both in order to get familiar with how this is done, and to get an idea of how much time will be needed for preparing the equipment at the time of recording. If time is short, this might be crucial to whether all parts of the investigated activity can be recorded.

Practical Guidelines for Preparation for Data Collection
- Apply for ethical approval in good time before the start of the project
- Permission to undertake the study must be obtained both from the management and the individuals that are to be recorded
- Prepare oral and written information about the project to be presented to the informants. Attach a separate counterfoil for written consent
- Visit the research site prior to recording in order to plan recording arrangements and equipment
- Test all recording equipment to get familiar with how it works and how much time will be needed for mounting it

3.2.2 Doing Data Collection

As part of the research project, each of the research groups video recorded interprofessional simulation training for health care students and professionals. The following two paragraphs will describe the procedures for informing about the project and obtaining informed consent, and for recording of the training.

3.2.2.1 Informing About the Project and Obtaining Informed Consent

Prior to the start of the simulation training, the researchers presented the project to the training participants. The presentation was based on the information sheet sent out in advance and supplemented with more detailed information on what would be studied, the intended contributions of the research, and how the data would be used, stored and presented. The participants were then given the opportunity to read through the information sheet and asked for written consent to be video recorded for the purpose of the research project. Most of the requested participants gave their approval, and only in a few occasions arrangements with groups not being video recorded were required.

As stressed by Heath et al. (2010) access to a setting is an ongoing concern. Consequently, informants not only need to approve participation initially, but for the research to proceed as planned they must also continue to be willing to participate. If informants start to feel uncomfortable with being video recorded, they might resist involvement in various ways. Not necessarily by withdrawing their consent, but for instance by trying to avoid the view of the camera, or by having conversations quietly or at a distance from the microphones (Heath et al. 2010, p. 16). Maintaining the trust and communication with informants should thus be a central concern for researchers undertaking video-based research, as well as being sensitive to any concerns related to the research.

3.2.2.2   Recording

To ensure that the simulation training could be video recorded from the start at each recording occasion, we made sure to be in place well before the participants arrived to prepare the recording equipment. In addition to the time aspect, mounting the equipment in an empty room is preferable for other reasons. Since this procedure typically requires some space it is easier to perform when the room is not crowded. Moreover, less attention is typically paid to the recording equipment if it is already in place than if the cameraperson/s is preparing it when the informants arrive.

As mentioned earlier the research teams tried as far as possible to plan positions and viewpoints of the cameras in advance. In order not to be forced to remain near the cameras during recording, we had planned to use fixed camera positions and single viewpoints encompassing as much as possible of the simulation activities. This worked as planned to a large extent, but in some cases, adjustments were needed. During the first recording occasion in the pilot study, for instance, we realized that it was not possible to obtain a sharp image of the video clips displayed at the projector screen without zooming, and likewise, zooming was necessary to distinguish the facilitators' written notes. As stressed by Heath et al. (2010, p. 44) it is important to consider how the presence of researchers and cameras affect the actions under study, especially if the researcher remains near the camera and actively maneuvers it. This question of whether and how being under observation influences the informants' behavior is a frequently raised one in video-based research contexts. A common assumption is that the presence of researchers and recording equipment will result in an "unnatural" behavior. Considering this issue, the following statement by Goodwin, an influential researcher in the field of video-based interaction studies, is useful:

> The issue of how participants deal with observation is in fact a subtle one. Within conversation, participants never behave as if they were unobserved; it is clear that they organize their behaviour in terms of the observation it will receive from their coparticipants. For example, a speaker does not simply "forget" a word; instead, he actively displays to the others present that he is searching for a word. Thus, the issue is, not what participants do when they are unobserved, but whether the techniques they use to deal with observation by a camera are different from those used to deal with observation by co-participants. (1981, p. 44)

As outlined in the above quote, being observed is not specific for individuals participating in research, but it is a ubiquitous feature of all social situations. The question is thus not *if* the informants are aware of being observed – because they certainly are – but rather if they, as a consequence of the presence of the researcher and the camera, do something they would not normally do when being observed by others. An argument here would be that this is difficult to determine for someone not familiar with how the recorded individuals normally behave. But as pointed out by Heath et al. (2010), however, a close examination of the recorded materials can help to reveal if the informants are orienting towards the camera or not. In the pilot study, the video recordings were reviewed after each recording occasion in order to, using the words of Heath et al. (2010), "find evidence of the participants orienting to the filming and if instances [were] found then consider how they [arose]and why" (p. 48). No such instances requiring adjustments of the recording routines were found, but as it appeared from the recordings the informants directed their attention towards the simulation activities rather than the cameras. Still, however, when recording in the research project, the research teams constantly sought to avoid drawing unnecessary attention towards the recording equipment. When not actively maneuvering the cameras, standing nearby them looking through the viewfinders was avoided, and instead the researchers tried to remain in the background to not interfere in the scene more than necessary.

Practical Guidelines for Doing Data Collection
- Provide information about the research and retrieve informed consent as early as possible to be able to start recording, but do not interfere with central routines of the setting
- Allocate some time for questions after the information and make sure to be sensitive to potential concerns of the participants related to the research
- Do not try to persuade anyone who does not want to participate, but if you suspect that the denial is due to misunderstandings, try to address those matters
- Check with the management if it is possible to organize the training in a way that enables recording of only some participants/groups so that it is possible to perform the study even if some individuals do not want to take part

3.2.3   After Data Collection

Preparations for and implementation of data collection is time consuming, and so is the post-processing of the recorded materials. In addition to the work of transferring the video recordings from camera to hard drive, and possible conversion to into more easy-to-use file formats, post-processing also includes storing and backup on safe and affordable storage areas. In the case of research materials, there are rules for how materials can be stored and how long the data shall be saved that researchers are required to follow. The following paragraphs describe how such issues were handled in the research project.

3.2.3.1 Post-processing of Recorded Material

An important implication derived from the pilot study was to transfer the video recordings from cameras/tapes to hard drive and do necessary post-processing of the video files after each recording occasion. This enabled for the researchers to identify possible shortcomings that required adjustments of the recording arrangements prior to upcoming recordings. The raw files, that is, the uncompressed video files, were stored on external hard drives locked into safes as backups of the video data. The compressed video files which would be used as basis for analyses were stored on password-protected external hard drives, which when not used were also stored in safes. In addition to prevent unauthorized persons from getting access to the video material, storage in a data media safe also provides some protection against fire and water leakage,[7] and is thus a necessity for safe storage of hard drives and tapes containing research data. However, while such storage can be regarded as a sufficient solution it is recommended that research materials, preferably with regard to costs and available infrastructure, are also stored at protected server spaces. At the time for the start of the project, however, server storage that met the requirements for storage of research data was very expensive. Therefore, it took a couple of years before this could arranged at all three sites.

Each recorded simulation activity was represented by a separate video file to enable the project members to get a clear overview of the video data as stored on disk. In the pilot study, a joint system for the naming of these video files was developed. The file name provided information on participant category (students or professionals), recording site, date of recording, type of activity (e.g. debriefing), and activity number (e.g. debriefing number three). For activities recorded with two cameras, an A or a B at the end of the file name gave information on what camera had been used for recording.

3.2.3.2 Sharing of Recorded Material

When data collection was complete, recordings of ten simulation sessions from each site were to be shared with the other research groups. Initially, this was meant to be done via a shared server space. As mentioned above however, we were not able to find a sufficiently affordable and safe solution. To ensure that unauthorized persons cannot get access to video data stored on a server, encryption of the files is required. At the time of the start of the research project, neither of the research group's home universities had access to a secure encryption solution which meant that this sharing method could not be used. As an alternative solution, we decided to use password-protected external hard drives to exchange video files in the project. Each research team purchased two password-protected external hard drives, on which the ten recordings to be shared with the other research teams were stored. These hard drives were then exchanged at a joint project meeting.

---

[7] A data media safe is designed to give better protection against heat, smoke and water than a regular safe.

Practical Guidelines for Post-processing of Data

- Review the recordings after each recording occasion to identify potential short-comings that require adjustments prior to the next recording occasion
- Create a separate video-file for each file for each recorded activity and name the files according to a uniform system to get a good overview of the video files as stored on hard drive
- If possible, purchase a safe server space for storage and backup of the video files. An alternative is storage on hard drives stored in a data media safe
- To prevent unauthorized access, always use password-protected hard drives for storage of research data that will be transported or kept outside a safe

3.2.4 Implementing a Common Method for Data Collection Across Different Sites

Experiences from the pilot study were continuously documented, and after its completion summarized into the guidelines presented above. These guidelines formed the basis for a joint workshop that was arranged at an early stage of the major research project. At the workshop, each phase of data collection was presented in detail, and the research teams were provided with a checklist comprising key issues of data collection. After the workshop, the project's shared documents, such as meeting notes, the checklist for data collection, the form for written information and informed consent, were uploaded on a shared server storage hosted by one of the research team's home university. As the project progressed, the shared server space constituted a collaboration area for the project members, enabling quick and easy exchange of information, publications and other documents.

References

Derry, S. J., Pea, R. D., Barron, B., Engle, R. A., Erickson, F., Goldman, R., & Sherin, B. L. (2010). Conducting video research in the learning sciences: Guidance on selection, analysis, technology, and ethics. *The Journal of the Learning Sciences, 19*(1), 3–53.

Goodwin, C. (1981). *Conversational organization: Interaction between speakers and hearers*. New York: Academic.

Heath, C., Hindmarsh, J., & Luff. P. (2010). *Video in qualitative research. Analysing social interaction in everyday life*. London: Sage.

Knoblauch, H., Schnettler, B., Raab, J., & Soeffner, H. G. (2006). *Video analysis: Methodology and methods. Qualitative audiovisual data analysis in sociology*. Frankfurt am Main: Peter Lang.

Koschmann, T., LeBaron, C., Goodwin, C., & Feltovich, P. (2011). "Can you see the cystic artery yet?": A simple matter of trust. *Journal of Pragmatics, 43*(2), 521–541.

Lindwall, O., Johansson, E., Rystedt, H., Ivarsson, J., & Reit, C. (2014). The use of video in dental education: Clinical reality addressed as practical matters of production, interpretation and instruction. In M. Broth, E. Laurier, & L. Mondada (Eds.), *Video at work. Praxeological studies of media production* (pp. 161–180). New York: Routledge.

Mondada, L. (2003). Working with video: How surgeons produce video recordings of their actions. *Visual Studies, 18*(1), 58–73.

Rystedt, H., & Sjöblom, B. (2012). Realism, authenticity, and learning in healthcare simulations: Rules of relevance and irrelevance as interactive achievement. *Instructional Science, 40*(5), 785–798.

Rystedt, H., Ivarsson, J., Asplund, S., Allansdotter Johnsson, Å., & Båth, M. (2011). Rediscovering radiology: New technologies and remedial action at the worksite. *Social Studies of Science, 41*(6), 867–891.

Sanchez Svensson, M., Luff, P., & Heath, C. (2009). Embedding instruction in practice: Contingency and collaboration during surgical training. *Sociology of Health & Illness, 31*(6), 889–906.

Vetenskapsrådet. (2017). God forskningssed. (Vetenskapsrådets rapportserie 1651–7350; 2011:1). Accessed 6 Sept 2017, from https://publikationer.vr.se/produkt/god-forskningssed/

3.3   Approaches to Analyzing Videodata

Madeleine Abrandt Dahlgren
Linköping University
Linköping, Sweden
e-mail: madeleine.abrandt.dahlgren@liu.se

Donna Rooney
University of Technology
Sydney, Australia
e-mail: donna.rooney@uts.edu.au

Hans Rystedt
University of Gothenburg
Gothenburg, Sweden
e-mail: hans.rystedt@ped.gu.se

This section will provide three examples of how video data can be analyzed from different perspectives. The examples illustrate how data analyses were organized within and across different sites and project groups. The first example is a purposeful approach to collaborative data analysis of interprofessional simulation-based practices that were developed within the SIMIPL research group. A practice theory perspective directs the analytical attention to how the nexus of actions hangs together through sayings, doings and relatings. The analysis comprises a layered process of constant comparisons, following three phases, moving from analysis of a single video recorded scenario, to the identification of patterns across recordings and scenarios. A second example from the SIMIPL project is based on video-based studies of situated action, an approach that draws on ethnomethodology (EM) and conversation analysis (CA). This approach puts the analytical focus on how participants in simulation activities are able to achieve and maintain shared understandings of events through talk, gestures and action in interaction with each other and the technical environment. This imply a scrutiny of how talk-in-interaction is sequentially organized, for instance the relation between questions and responses in the debriefings (Sect. 7.3).

A third example is a collaborative analysis is the use of qualitatively different readings of the same video data, that was developed within the research group at UTS. One does not replace the other, but rather draws out different features. They arrive at a view that represents the most significant shift away from accounts found in existing literature. The readings share the same empirical reference point, and a consistent theoretical basis, grounded in practice theory.

In this section, we will showcase examples of how collaborative analyses of data have been carried out.

3.3.1 Perspectives on Video Data Analysis

Typically, the methodological issues raised in relation to the use of video as a method of data collection have concerned technical aspects such as placement and angles of cameras, as well as issues of access to record, ethical issues and the possible effect of video recording on the on-going activities (Luff and Heath 2012). The use of video is also claimed to require thoughtful considerations relating to all stages of the research process. Initially, decisions such as the ones described in Sect. 3.2, regarding the site for the video recordings, the focus, time and duration of the film are necessary. These aspects are important, not the least in relation to considerations about theoretical frameworks and focus for the research. What fragments for analysis from the corpus of data should be selected, how should data be transcribed and categorized? The theoretical framework, the applied analysis and the collected material need to resonate (Luff and Heath 2012), just as in any other research approach. The authors point to the fact that the use of video as a means of data collection in qualitative research has not been subject to discussions of methodological concerns to the same extent that more traditional methods, such as interviews, fieldwork or focus groups. The use of collaborative data analysis of video-data in simulation-based education is probably even more seldomly described. Methodological considerations are generally viewed as adamant in order to obtain quality in any research. Criteria for judging the quality of qualitative research have been discussed by several authors (e.g. Seale 1999, 2002; Larsson 2005; Hammersley 2007; Polit and Beck 2014). However, due to the diverse and manifold of approaches to qualitative research, there is no general consensus on how to assess quality in qualitative research. Quality criteria for qualitative research based on methodological issues are often referred to as trustworthiness and address the rigor of the study (Polit and Beck 2014), i.e. to what extent methods, data and interpretations can be trusted and ensure the quality of a study (Polit and Beck 2014). Such criteria have been outlined by Lincoln and Guba (1985). Connelly (2016) summarizes these criteria as concerning *credibility*, i.e. the confidence in the truth of the findings; *dependability*, i.e. the stability of the data over time and over the conditions of the study; *confirmability*, i.e. to what extent findings are consistent and could be repeated, and *transferability*, i.e. to what extent the findings are applicable to other settings; and *authenticity*, i.e. to what extent the researchers can provide a realistic, rich and detailed description of the participants and settings studied. In addition to quality aspects regarding methodological rigor of qualitative research that are important and adamant in any research, there are also criteria for judging the quality of conceptualization of the study, and interpretations of findings in addition to the methodological and analytical considerations. Larsson (2005) suggests that these criteria can be summarized as a concern for perspective awareness, internal consistency and ethical considerations of the work as a whole, and also the quality of the findings. Larsson (2005) suggest that the quality of the findings could be judged according to three criteria, i.e. the richness of meaning, the structure of presentation of the findings, and the extent to which the findings contribute to theory development. Embedded in the judgement of quality of the research as a whole are also five validity criteria, according to Larsson (2005). These concern whether the research is convincing in the discourse of the research community as a disciplined inquiry, and whether the research enables the reader to see a phenomenon in a new way. Further, the research should display a sound empirical anchoring of findings, and a discernible consistency between the overall interpretation and the constituent empirical data. Finally, the research should address the 'so what' question to fulfil a pragmatic criterion of validity, i.e. the value and implications of the research for practice (Larsson 2005).

3.3.2   Purposeful Approach to Collaborative Data Analysis

For our first example of analysis of video-data, we will describe a purposeful approach to collaborative data analysis, comprising a layered process in three phases of activities. The process was developed by the collaborating research teams of the SIMIPL project (Nyström et al. 2016; Escher et al. 2017). The teams were inspired by constant comparative analysis as described by Boeije (2002), the zooming in and out as an approach to theorizing work and organizational practices as described by Nicolini (2009) and video analysis as described by Heath et al. (2010). The video-data comprised various simulation scenarios, that were enacted by different interprofessional teams of undergraduate nursing and medical students as part of their educational programs, or of professional nurses and physicians, participating in simulation training as part of continuing educational development activities. The collected video-recordings made up a common pool of empirical data that was shared and subject to different analyses, individual as well as collaborative, across the members of the research team. In the following, we will give an account of the phases of collaborative data analysis, their respective purposes and activities to answer specific questions were developed. We will also discuss the results of each phase, how the preliminary findings led to decisions about focus and process for further analysis.

3.3.2.1 Phase 1. Comparisons of Multiple Views of a Single Video-Recording

The purpose of the first phase of the analysis was to develop a collectively enriched and shared understanding of what was happening in the enactment of the sequence of activities in the simulation scenario. The research group watched the video together, taking individual field notes as the scenario was played out. The note taking was guided by common analytical questions, that helped the researchers to zoom in on and make certain aspects of the simulation practice become foregrounded (Nicolini 2009), in our case, e.g. how different professional knowings were made relevant in the debriefing of the simulation (Nyström et al. 2016) or how scenario information that could not be conveyed through the simulator was provided by facilitators as described by Escher et al. (2017). Nyström et al. describe how a first round of comparisons, the individual notes were negotiated and merged, assisting the researchers in reaching consensus on interpretations of the fragments observed. As a result of the first phase, the focus for further zooming in was specified, e.g. to the openings, interaction and closing of the debriefing.

3.3.2.2 Phase 2. Comparisons Between Different Recordings of the Same or a Similar Scenario

The purpose of the second phase was to identify patterns re-occurring across the data, and to develop a shared understanding these. In this phase, the common analytical questions were zooming out to theorize how socio-material arrangements were related to sayings and doings in the debriefing, comparing openings, interactions, closings and the interconnections between human and non-human actors across several video-recordings of the same or similar scenario, enacted by different teams of participants. Sequences were selected across the data and transcribed. Provisional interpretations of the patterns identified in the debriefing, relational to e.g. structure/lack of structure was formulated as a focus for a third round of analyses and comparisons.

3.3.2.3 Phase 3. Comparison Between Video Recordings of Different Scenarios

The purpose of the third round of analysis was to zoom out in order to enlarge and enrich the basis for interpretation of how through identifying the variation and similarities in how debriefing of interprofessional collaboration is enacted. Through the zooming out, the provisional interpretations were refined against wider data and theory. The process of analysis thus follows what Nicolini (2009) describes as a *"double movement of zooming in on and zooming out of practice obtained by switching theoretical lenses and following or trailing the connections between practices"* (p. 1392).

It has been pointed out that in order to understand the captured fragments of the ongoing activity, it might be important to also bring in the participants' perspectives (Luff and Heath 2012). The use of video as a means of data collection should therefore preferably also be accompanied by ethnographic fieldwork and interviews. The video recordings can then fulfil a double purpose, both as a means of collecting data, and as a means of stimulus for interview with participants, who can explain how the captured video data fit into the bigger picture of the activity studied. Hopwood (2014) showed that the use of video as a stimulus prompted the participants reflections and comments. In our case, the work situation we are studying is an arranged in such a way that the sequence of events is very clearly structured, following the pre-defined steps of briefing, simulation and debriefing. The briefing takes place beforehand of what is going to happen, i.e. the upcoming scenario, and the debriefing takes place *post factum,* where the participants reflect on the events, actions and interactions that emerged in the simulation scenario. This structure has been helpful for the team of researchers to understand the video-recorded situations and some of the 'back stage' activities and arrangements, even if the bulk of our data are observational. In addition to the observations, informal and in some cases also formal interviews with the instructors have been conducted in order to complement the observational data.

The theoretical perspective directed the analytical attention towards how the nexus of actions hanged together as relationships between material entities including both human actors, such as bodies, and non-human actors, such as the arrangements of patients' and students' bodies, clinical environments, and protocols in use (Nyström et al. 2016). In other words, the focus on the interplay between participants and the physical environment.

3.3.3   Video-Based Studies on Situated Action

As presented in Sect. 2.2, this analytical approach is informed by ethnomethodology (EM) and conversation analysis (CA): two closely intertwined perspectives with an interest in how social order and intersubjective understandings are constituted and maintained through talk-in-interaction (Garfinkel 1967; Sacks 1992). The organization of such an order includes embodied and material aspects, implying that it is the participants' interactions in the material surround that is of primarily analytical concern (e.g. Eikeland Husebø et al. 2012; Johansson et al. 2017). However, the interest for intricate details of the participants' interactions, and the extensive amounts of video data to be analysed, calls for systematic methods for data management, retrieval and selection (Knoblauch et al. 2006).

3.3.3.1   Reviewing, Cataloguing and Selecting Data

In our research, we have followed a three-step review of the entire video material suggested by Heath et al. (2010). The first step includes a *preliminary review* in form of systematic coding of the whole data corpus, or alternatively, a time-stamped content log of key events (Derry et al. 2010) to get an overview of the data corpus and possibilities to find and revisit and compare interesting parts. Secondly, a more *substantive review* involves repeated reviews of the particular activities that are identified as interesting by the research group. In the case of Sect. 7.3, for instance, the way the instructors designed their questions during debriefings emerged as an interesting phenomenon for further investigation. In a third step, the *analytic review*, repeated reviews of related data sets were conducted to find instances of actions that seemed to display similar characteristics and create collections of episodes for further analysis. In the case of Sect. 7.3, the participants' explicit references to audio-visual features of video-clips of scenarios were identified as a topic for further analysis and comprised a collection. Such collections, in turn, constituted the primary data for the analysis by allowing us to compare and contrast how activities were carried out under different circumstances. An essential part of the analysis process was to review data in the research group to discuss preliminary observations and develop ideas for further investigations. In addition, selections of video data deemed as particularly interesting were presented in joint data sessions arranged by the Network for Analyses of Interaction and Learning (NAIL) at the University of Gothenburg. During these sessions, collaborative and detailed analyses of brief sequences were performed, primarily in the spirit of ethnomethodology and conversation analysis.

3.3.3.2   Transcription

Transcription is an indispensable part of the analysis, since it is not just a way of representing audiovisual data. As pointed out by Knoblauch et al. (2006): "Transcribing generates observations that are fundamental to analytical inferences" (p. 16). Since transcribing all data on a detailed level is far too time-consuming, only the instances selected for closer investigation were transcribed on that level. These transcripts mainly followed a system that was originally developed by Jefferson (1984). This system is motivated by an interest in the sequential organization of talk-in-interaction; how participants take turns and the significance of conversational features such as overlap, pauses, emphasis, intonation, loud/low talk, cut of, laughter etc. A detailed presentation of these conventions can be found in Sect. 7.3. Further, participants' non-verbal actions available via video recordings were added to the transcripts if these were deemed as consequential for understanding the organization of the analyzed interactions. As shown in Sect. 4.2, for instance, the participants' gaze and bodily positions play a significant role for how they were able to achieve a shared understanding of how a given task should be carried out in the simulation environment. It is important to note however, that the transcript in itself is not the basis for the analysis, but primarily function as a means for refining the analysis. Therefore, the original video recordings were regularly revisited to get access to details of interaction that were not represented by the transcription as such.

3.3.3.3 Reliability and Validity

Similar to other qualitative methods, ethnomethodology and conversation analysis share the ambition to produce descriptions that in some controllable way correspond to the social world that is investigated. Although all such descriptions are theory dependent, and necessarily represent social worlds in different ways, it is still possible to provide accounts that can be exposed to empirical testing and, thereby to meet demands on reliability and validity. Reliability does to a large extent rely on the inclusiveness and quality of the recordings. The measures developed by the research group to meet these demands are extensively presented and discussed in Sect. 3.2.

With respect to validity, one ambition of particular concern in our studies on situated action, was to strengthen the validity of interpretations through the *proof procedure* described by Sacks et al. (1974). Considered in isolation, all utterances could be seen as more or less open ended. As shown by studies of talk-in-interaction, however, utterances in conversation are organized in such way that each successive utterance provides the conditions for the production of a relevant next. For instance, questions project answers, offers project acceptances or declinations etc. The next utterance, in turn, builds on displays an understanding of the prior. A response in the form of an acceptance shows that the prior utterance was understood as an offer. First and foremost, this order is central for to the progression of talk, but it also provides the researcher with a proof criterion for the analysis of talk. The criterion for validity from this point of view is that the next turn will display whether or not the participants themselves threat an utterance in a way that is in line with the interpretation of the analyst. Another ambition, in line with the proof procedure, was that claims on the *institutional character* of activities have to substantiated by the ways the participants themselves orient to such features. Consequently, it is not sufficiently to state that a certain type of behaviour is the result of certain institutional characteristics, for instance that the activities under scrutiny are caused by certain institutional norms (Drew and Heritage 1992). Instead we have sought to unpack how the participants themselves visibly orient to and make such norms relevant in their interactions. In striving for this, we have tried to unravel the significance of institutional order by the ways it is invoked by the participants.

In all, the quest for meeting these criteria on validity is quite demanding and requires extensive experiences of analysing video recorded interactions. Therefore, the joint NAIL seminars at the university constituted an invaluable resource for testing preliminary interpretations and strengthening the credibility of the analytical claims.

3.3.4 Qualitatively Different Readings of the Same Data

Like the Swedish research presented throughout this volume, the data collection methods used by Australian researchers with a similar project were ethnographic in nature and well suited to empirical study of practices (Schatzki 2012, p. 25). The multidisciplinary team observed, videoed and audio recorded ten simulation events (Rooney et al. 2015). The simulation lab consists of three different spaces; a 'normal' classroom with a lectern, student desks, chairs, and a screen; another space with a hospital bed, and an array of hospital equipment (e.g. monitors, trolleys, hospital bed and manikin etc.) separated from the first via a partition; and, a third space consisting of a control room where a technician remotely controls the manikin as well as the relays video of bedside action to the students as observers in the traditional classroom space. In each simulation class 3–4 researchers were positioned across these different spaces, enabling each to focus observations on different activities within the class: e.g. bedside, control room, and observing students' activities. Researchers made unstructured field notes as well as audio recordings of the 'talk' occurring in the space they were observing and, what is of particular importance to this section, the simulation classes were filmed from various locations.

These methods accrued a rich data set: in addition to 85 pages of text and approximately 24 pages of drawings and other non-text field notes, our methods accrued 598 min of audio recordings and 493 min of video. Here we focus on how the team analyzed the later (i.e. video).

3.3.4.1 Individual and Parallel Readings: Productive Pluralism

As a starting point each team member was allocated 2–3 videos to watch in closer detail: with each of the videos being viewed by at least two team members. Aspects of the video could be clarified by accessing transcripts or field notes relating to the same simulation when necessary. The agreed instructions for the team were simply to identify moments that were pedagogically interesting – while "interesting" was not pre-defined, the team agreed to document why they judged them to be so. A template (see Table 3.1) was created so individual researchers could document their "moments" with a view to share and discuss these with the team.

Productive pluralism (Frost et al. 2010) enriched the interrogation of the data as the individual interests informed what struck each as interesting. For instance, in the example below three interesting moments are identified by three different researchers. However, note that the third column shows that these moments occurred at more or less the same time. Yet the justifications offered by each of the researchers (in the second column) are framed in various ways; novice nurse practice; 'reality'; space; activities; and, materiality.

Table 3.1 Template for documenting observations

What is happening?	Why is this interesting?	Where can we find it?
2nd nurse focused on oxygen readings from the monitor – stops questioning patient and looks for the other mask	Highlights typical novice practice – seeking to do or act (single task) rather than continuing discussions with the manikin. Does this mean manikin $\neq$ reality OR would the student do similar with a real person?	VIDEO: 130819 Sim 2_3_5 Start >1:20
First, actor on the left adjusts sim man's shirt, and later his mask. Actor on right looks at 'him' while explaining pains in chest and motions chest toward him (as if 'real')– then however, twice quickly after the actor on right goes through motions of taking pulse (?) without actually 'really doing it' – there is a quick touch but not nurse-like activity	Because the manikin is both 'real' and 'unreal'? – perhaps the actor is working in a sort of betwixt space	VIDEO: 130819 Sim 2_3_5 1:09 > 1:17
When change rebreather, take off glasses, nurse looks up at screen and also feels for pulse	Really materially engaged in the material and clinical world of Ken	VIDEO: 130819 Sim 2_3_5 about 1:35

Table 3.2 Template for documenting observations

What is happening?	Why is this interesting?	Where can we find it?
Start changing mask over, girlfriend reaches out to sim man – honey are you ok? 2 nurses v materially engaged (third one still standing doing/saying nothing as per most of sim)	Again the material engagement – particularly girlfriend reaching out to sim man; she stays holding him for ages	VIDEO: 130819 Sim2_3_5. around 8:45 130,819 raw notes DR – seem to be some z-z z-z [code used for disengaged

3.3.4.2 Multiple Video Recordings of the Same Classroom

With multiple video recordings of the same classroom available (viewed in conjunction with other data sources), readings of the different classroom spaces at the same point in time were possible. For instance, an identified moment of student-nurses being materially engaged in the simulation was positioned alongside disengaged student observers (see Table 3.2).

The result of our analysis was a multiplicity of moments within the simulation videos that were pedagogically interesting for various reasons. This axial work (Boeije 2002) enabled the team to formulate criteria for comparison, sharpen their collective understanding of simulation pedagogy. The analytical pastiche raised new questions about the fluidity of fidelity in a simulation classroom (e.g. *What is being simulated?*), as well as provided insight into the interplay of its human and non-human actors.

3.3.4.3 Refining Layered Readings

The multiplicity of interesting moments was gradually refined into a number of layered readings, as varied theoretical tools were applied, and their application sharpened through a consensual, although not reductive, layering strategy (Rooney et al. 2015). The aim was not one of 'gladiator' scholarship (Rojeck 1998, p. 12), i.e. to annihilate the established framing of simulation for a superior practice-based version. Rather, like the divergent readings of the videos, the team produced conceptual understandings in order to raise new sorts of questions. Also like the layered 'readings' of the rich data set, a layering of understandings (inclusive of practice based *and* established framings) were provided in the publication where differences sat together in unresolved contention: 'pedagogically interesting' in its own right (Rooney et al. 2015).

3.4 Conclusions

The purpose of introducing different approaches to analyses of video-data in this chapter was to bring about a discussion of how different theoretical and methodological approaches to the analyses of video-recorded data of interprofessional simulation-based healthcare education can contribute to an enriched understanding of the phenomenon. The three empirical examples presented are all focusing on practice, but the theoretical frameworks and approaches to analyses differ. The researchers themselves represent different professions, practitioners and educators that contribute their expertise and unique understanding to the analysis. The issue of how different theoretical perspectives framing the examples highlight different aspects of similar phenomena, thereby offering approaches to research that can, taken together, enrich our understanding of interprofessional simulation as an educational practice.

References

Boeije, H. (2002). A purposeful approach to the constant comparative method in the analysis of qualitative interviews. *Quality and Quantity, 36*, 391–409.

Connelly, L. M. (2016). Trustworthiness in qualitative research. *MEDSURG Nursing, 25*(6), 435–436.

Derry, S. J., Pea, R. D., Barron, B., Engle, R. A., Erickson, F., Goldman, R., et al. (2010). Conducting video research in the learning sciences: Guidance on selection, analysis, technology, and ethics. *The Journal of the Learning Sciences, 19*(1), 3–53. https://doi.org/10.1080/10508400903452884.

Drew, P., & Heritage, J. (1992). *Talk at work: Interaction in institutional settings.* Cambridge: Cambridge University Press.

Eikeland Husebø, S., Friberg, F., Søreide, E., & Rystedt, H. (2012). Instructional problems in briefings: How to prepare nursing students for simulation-based cardiopulmonary resuscitation training. *Clinical Simulation in Nursing, 8*(7), e307–e318. https://doi.org/10.1016/j.ecns.2010.12.002.

Escher, C., Rystedt, H., Creutzfeldt, J., Meurling, L., Nyström, S., Dahlberg, J., et al. (2017). Method matters: Impact of in-scenario instruction on simulation-based teamwork training. *Advances in Simulation, 2*(1), 1–8.

Frost, N., Nolas, S. M., Brooks-Gordon, B., Esin, C., Holt, A., Mehdizadeh, L., & Shinebourne, P. (2010). Pluralism in qualitative research: The impact of different researchers and qualitative approaches on the analysis of qualitative data. *Qualitative   Research,   10*(4),   441–460.   https://doi. org/10.1177/1468794110366802.

Garfinkel, H. (1967). *Studies in ethnomethodology.* Englewood Cliffs: Prentice-Hall.

Hammersley, M. (2007). The issue of quality in qualitative research. *International Journal of Research & Method in Education, 30*(3), 287–305.

Heath, C., Hindmarsh, J., & Luff. P. (2010). *Video in qualitative research. Analysing social interaction in everyday life.* London: Sage.

Hopwood, N. (2014). Using video to trace the embodied and material in a study of health practice. *Qualitative Research Journal, 14*(2), 197–211.

Jefferson, G. (1984). Transcript notation. In M. Atkinson & J. Heritage (Eds.), *Structures of social action* (pp. ix–xvi). New York: Cambridge University Press.

Johansson, E., Lindwall, O., & Rystedt, H. (2017). Experiences, appearances, and interprofessional training: The instructional use of video in post-simulation debriefings. *International Journal of Computer-Supported Collaborative Learning, 12*(1), 91–112. https://doi.org/10.1007/s11412-017-9252-z

Knoblauch, H., Schnettler, B., Raab, J., & Soeffner, H. G. (2006). *Video analysis: Methodology and methods. Qualitative audiovisual data analysis in sociology.* Frankfurt am Main: Peter Lang.

Larsson, S. (2005). Om kvalitet i kvalitativa studier [On quality in qualitative research]. *Nordisk Pedagogik, 25*(1), 16–35.

Lincoln, Y. S., & Guba, E. G. (1985) *Naturalistic inquiry.* Newbury Park: Sage.

Luff, P., & Heath, C. (2012). Some 'technical challenges' of video analysis: Social actions, objects, material realities and the problems of perspective. *Qualitative Research, 12*(3), 255–279.

Nicolini, D. (2009). Zooming in and out: Studying practices by switching theoretical lenses and trailing connections. *Organization, 30*(12), 1391–1418.

Nyström, S., Dahlberg, J., Hult, H., & Abrandt Dahlgren, M. (2016). Observing of interprofessional collaboration in simulation: A socio-material approach. *Journal of Interprofessional Care, 30*(6), 710–716.

Polit, D. F., & Beck, C. T. (2014) *Essentials of nursing research: Appraising evidence for nursing practice* (8th ed.). Philadelphia: Wolters Kluwer/Lippincott Williams & Wilkins.

Rojeck, C. (1998). Lyotard and the decline of 'society'. In C. Rojeck (Ed.), *Politics of Jean-Francois Lyotard* (pp. 10–19). London: Routledge.

Rooney, D., Hopwood, N., Boud, D., & Kelly, M. (2015). The role of simulation in pedagogies of higher education for the health professions: Through a practice-based lens. *Vocations and Learning, 8*, 269–285. https://doi.org/10.1007/s12186-015-9138-z.

Sacks, H. (1992). *Lectures on conversation, vol. I & II* (Edited by G. Jefferson with an introduction by E. A. Schegloff). Oxford: Basil Blackwell.

Sacks, H., Schegloff, E. A., & Jefferson, G. (1974). A simplest systematics for the organization of turn-taking for conversation. *Language, 50*(4), 696–735.

Schatzki, T. (2012). A primer on practices. In J. Higgs, R. Barnett, S. Billett, M. Hutchings, & F. Trede (Eds.), *Practice-based education: Perspectives and strategies* (pp. 13–26). Rotterdam: Sense Publishers.

Seale, C. (1999). *The quality of qualitative research*. London: Sage.

Seale, C. (2002). Quality issues in qualitative inquiry. *Qualitative Social Work, 1*(1), 97–110.

Part II
The Practices of Interprofessional Simulation – Preparing, Doing, Observing and Reflecting

Chapter 4
Preparing for Team Work Training in Simulation

Michelle Kelly, Sissel Eikeland Husebø, Hans Rystedt, Cecilia Escher, Johan Creutzfeldt, Lisbet Meurling, Li Felländer-Tsai, and Håkan Hult

4.1 Introduction

Michelle Kelly
Curtin University
Perth, Australia
email: michelle.kelly@curtin.edu.au

Working together, within and across health disciplines, requires understanding of one's own and other professions' roles and contributions to patient management. Becoming nuanced in one's own practice has previously been the approach to becoming a health practitioner. However, this approach does not reflect the expectations of practice where teamwork and effective communication within and across disciplines is crucial to efficiencies, and desired patient outcomes. Over recent decades, there has been a concerted effort to promote opportunities to learn about

M. Kelly
Curtin University, Perth, Australia
e-mail: michelle.kelly@curtin.edu.au

S. E. Husebø (✉)
University of Stavanger, Stavanger, Norway
e-mail: sissel.i.husebo@uis.no

H. Rystedt
University of Gothenburg, Gothenburg, Sweden
e-mail: hans.rystedt@ped.gu.se

C. Escher · J. Creutzfeldt · L. Meurling · L. Felländer-Tsai · H. Hult
Karolinska Institutet, Stockholm, Sweden
e-mail: cecilia.escher@ki.se; johan.creutzfeldt@ki.se; lisbet.meurling@ki.se; li.tsai@ki.se; hakan.hult@ki.se

© Springer Nature Switzerland AG 2019
M. Abrandt Dahlgren et al. (eds.), *Interprofessional Simulation in Health Care*,
Professional and Practice-based Learning 26,
https://doi.org/10.1007/978-3-030-19542-7_4

and with other health professionals. This can be challenging given the differing work or study schedules. However, given the rise and popularity of simulation-based education (SBE), there is opportunity right from the outset in preparatory healthcare programs to reflect how teams can and should work together in practice.

In this chapter, about designing and facilitating teamwork training, a light is shone on two important aspects of SBE in this context: instructional challenges in designing scenarios, including preparing and facilitating learners in simulations; and approaches to maximize "non-technical" skills capabilities within authentic simulation scenarios.

To start, Husebø and Rystedt bring our attention to important aspects in preparing learners for simulations about patient resuscitation. Although they focus on novice learners, their concepts of students claiming an understanding verses exhibiting an understanding of practices is equally applicable to clinicians across all professions. There is much support in wider literature for modelling ideal practices, particularly for novice students or clinicians (essentially a Community of Practice) where learning can be scaffolded within meaningful contexts and applied to practice. The authors offer numerous examples from their research about instructional strategies to ensure novices become attuned to the nuances of practice, specifically when working within teams in a critically important aspect of patient care – resuscitation. Creating a shared understanding from the outset of what is expected from participating in the simulation activities is a highlighted feature of this section.

Similarly, Escher et al. focus on the criticality of 'non-technical' skills in interprofessional simulations, specifically how to maximize authenticity in relation to the learners' level of experience. In addition to providing useful frameworks from aviation for communicating in teams, the authors highlight the importance of the facilitator's role in SBE. Along with monitoring the simulation action, the facilitator can add an appropriate level of complexity to the unfolding scenario, to align with actual clinical situations and hence boost authenticity. In consideration of the participants' experience, and professional background, the facilitator is in a key position to promote the team's awareness of the differing discourses across professions. This alone can boost the fidelity of the simulation scenario, where a shared understanding of what is said and the impact of (mis)communication are featured learning outcomes. Clarity of message to match intent is particularly important feature of interprofessional simulations.

4.2   Instructional Challenges in Preparing for Simulation

Sissel Eikeland Husebø
University of Stavanger
Stavanger, Norway
email: sissel.i.husebo@uis.no

Hans Rystedt
University of Gothenburg
Gothenburg, Sweden
email: hans.rystedt@ped.gu.se

An important condition for serving the educational objectives of simulation-based team training in undergraduate nursing education is that the participants understand how clinical procedures should be performed in the situation the simulation is intended to represent. This subsection un-packs instructional challenges in briefings aimed at preparing undergraduate nursing students for performing resuscitation teamwork in subsequent scenarios. Whilst the teams in this empirical case can be seen as uniprofessional, it also highlights the challenges involved in assessing and furthering students' understanding of how to perform and coordinate individual tasks in interprofessional teamwork. The analytical focus is put on how instructors make use of students' exhibited understanding of tasks to demonstrate how these should be both performed and adapted to the specific conditions of the simulation.

4.2.1   What Do We Know About the Briefing Part of Simulation?

There is slightly different understanding of the notion of briefing. The following definition is commonly used: The noun "briefing" means "fact or situation of giving preliminary instruction" and is defined as "an activity immediately preceding the start of a simulation activity where the participants receive essential information about the simulation scenario, such as background information, vital signs, instructions, or guidelines" (Lopreiato et al. 2016, p. 6). In general, the purpose of the briefing is to set the stage for a scenario, assist participants in achieving scenario objectives, to establish a psychologically safe environment for participants, and to conduct the briefing as realistically as possible (Dieckmann 2009; Lopreiato et al. 2016). The briefing is described in several simulation textbooks (Bailey et al. 2010; Dieckmann 2009; Nestel et al. 2018). Nestel and Gough (2018) state that orientation to the learners are important and will include explicit discussion on what is similar and what is different to reality. An equal description is found in Bailey et al. (2010) who note that learners in the briefing are instructed as to which procedures can or cannot be performed on the mannequin, how to execute these procedures, and how these are different from those performed on a human being. Dieckmann (2009) put emphasis on that participants got to know the simulator and the simulated environment through explanations, demonstrations and hands-on time. He underlines that the participants must learn how to use the simulator, what is considered "normal" e.g. auscultation sounds of the manikin which are different from those of a "normal" patient due to mechanical noise. If the participants do not have sufficient competence to use the simulator as a tool, they may question its realism instead of the learning experience.

Despite the importance of participant preparation before onset of the simulation scenario, the briefing has rarely been explored (Husebø 2012; Nestel et al. 2018). Therefore, we conducted a review of the literature back to 2008, in January 2018, in the databases Academic Search Elite, CINAHL, Medline, and ERIC with the keywords briefing + simulation + health care. Of the 37 found, 18 studies were identified as relevant. Of those, eight studies contained a description of the briefing outlining ground rules for communication, methodology, educational objectives, simulation scenario, roles of the participants, examination of the manikin and equipment in the room (Arafeh et al. 2010; Bartlett et al. 2014; Bogossian et al. 2014; Calhoun et al. 2014; Kolbe et al. 2015; Koo et al. 2014; Morrison and Catanzaro 2010). Additionally, Kolbe et al. (2015) refer to Rudolph and colleagues (2014) who suggested a way for establishing a "safe container" in the briefing including clarifying expectations, establishing a fiction contract with trainers, explaining logistic details and respect and safety for the participants. Only two studies emphasized the briefing in the results (Beard 2013; Kelly et al. 2014). Kelly et al. (2014) found that the briefing did not receive very high ratings from nursing students for contributing to clinical judgment, while in Beard (2013) the learners perceive they would benefit from being prepared for the learning experience in the form of a pre-briefing. Only one empirical study was found that demonstrates the importance of the facilitator's instruction in the briefing for the nursing students' understanding of how they should perform in the simulation, how it is specifically related to the simulator, and what differences exists between the simulation environment and clinical practice (Husebø et al. 2012).

According to prevailing guidelines, the facilitator is responsible for the implementation and/or delivery of simulation activities, including the briefing (INACSL 2016a; Lopreiato et al. 2016) and responsible for managing the entire simulation-based experience. Still, research is scarce on how the facilitator's instructions could aid novice learners to perform tasks in simulation environments that they are mainly unfamiliar with. However, the significance of instructions has been addressed in qualitative sociological studies on simulation practice in medicine, nursing, dentistry and allied educations (Escher et al. 2017; Hindmarsh et al. 2014; Husebø et al. 2011; Johansson et al. 2017; Johnson 2007; Rystedt and Sjöblom 2012). Already in 2007, in the work done by Johnson (2007), it was demonstrated that the facilitators employed a wide range of instructional methods to bridge the gap between simulation and practice by for example reconstituting the patient's body and the facilitator's use of the own body as a metaphor for orientating the simulation to the conditions of medical practice. The facilitator also employed talk and gestures for reconstituting the simulation as a kind of medical practice. One implication of these results is that the simulations' relevance for learning is highly dependent on the facilitators' instruction. Although Escher and colleagues (2017) did not study the briefing in particular, they examined the variation of methods employed by facilitators in the simulation scenarios. The results demonstrate that facilitators' extra scenario information was essential for bridging the gap between the appearance of a sick patient and a manikin. Further, facilitators' close access to the teams' activities was critical for providing timely instructions and maintaining the flow of activities in the scenario. In dental education, Hindmarsh et al. (2014) studied how training with simulators was organized in and through tutor-student interaction. The findings emphasized the ways in which tutors routinely invoke real clinical practice in instructional corrections to compensate for the 'chronic insufficiency' of the simulator. However, the differences between clinical practice and simulators were also used to highlight aspects of the 'curriculum' that novice students had not yet experienced and thus could not master.

The research outlined above demonstrate that there is lack of studies focusing on briefing of interprofessional simulation. However, the few studies that was found in our review outlined above, demonstrate that the instructional corrections and the work that facilitators undertake to compensate for the "chronic insufficiency" of the simulator is essential for demonstrating how actions should be performed in the simulation session. Against this background, we will now turn to briefings and an empirical investigation of how performance of tasks and coordinated actions involved in all concerted teamwork could be assessed and demonstrated. Further, we will explore how the simulation environment function as a means for making the students' gaps in understanding visible and correctable. Of specific interest is:

1. how facilitators in and through instructions in the briefing make visible the practical skills necessary for nursing students to act in the simulation scenario
2. how students display their understandings of these skills
3. how facilitators make use of the students' claimed and exhibited understandings for correcting their performance

4.2.2 Setting and Analytic Approach

This section is based on video data from a study of teams consisting of three nursing students performing cardiopulmonary resuscitation (CPR) on a manikin in nursing education. The study took place in a simulation centre in the south-western part of Norway. The simulation localities resemble a patient room in a rehabilitation unit in a nursing home. A manikin positioned in a standard hospital bed represents the patient. The manikin was a "stand in" for an old woman with a history of angina pectoris who would suffer a cardiac arrest. Prior to the briefing, the students attended a 2-h lecture and a 1-h individual skills training session in the Norwegian guidelines for CPR and defibrillation (NNR 2015). The CPR and defibrillation guidelines had also been trained individually in each year of the nursing program. During the briefing, which lasted approximately 20 min, the facilitators gave each group an introduction concerning the functioning of the bed, the manikin and the medical equipment in the simulation room. The nursing students were instructed as to which procedures could or could not be performed on the manikin, how to execute these procedures, how these were different from those performed on a human being and how to use the medical devices during the scenario. The learning objectives of the simulation addressed by the facilitator during the briefing were to train the application of the CPR guidelines in teamwork and leadership. All objectives were part of the students' last clinical practice. In the following simulation scenarios, the teams comprised three students, one of whom was selected to be the team leader, the two others as assisting nurses. The three remaining students in each group and the facilitator were present in the room and observed the simulation. After one simulation they changed roles.

The analytic approach of this study is interaction analysis (IA), which has its roots in ethnomethodology and conversation analysis (Garfinkel 1967; Have 2007; Sacks et al. 1992). IA is a method for studying how people interact with each other and with the artifacts they have available in the environment. Its' objective is to identify how the participants' make their actions intelligible for one another and display their understanding of the actions of others (Heath et al. 2010; see also Sect. 2.2, this volume). The analyses follow the three steps suggested by Heath et al. (2010) and were partly subjected to collaborative analyses as presented in Sect. 3.3, this volume. First, all the video recordings from the briefings were reviewed. Second, the video recordings were reviewed with focus on events in the interaction between the facilitator and the nursing students. Third, the data corpus was undertaken for further analysis. The briefing examples were transcribed in detail by marking the facilitators' and nursing students' glances in relation to the conversation and gestures. As the analysis progressed, we identified recurrent patterns in the facilitators' instructions and the nursing students' response to these instructions.

4.2.3   Instructional Problems

We identified two types tasks that were especially problematic for the students to understand and master, which were addressed by facilitators in the briefings: "Taking the team leader's position" and "Keeping airways open". Both tasks are intertwined and critical for achieving successful resuscitation. Whilst, the first one mainly presupposes the coordination of teamwork, the second one necessities individual skills. These tasks created an instructional challenge in terms of demonstrating in a short time span the management of both equipment and simulator and monitoring if the students' understood how to act in the following scenario. Although the students had performed training earlier on resuscitation in their nursing program, the task on how to coordinate the teamwork and how to use the medical equipment were new for them.

4.2.3.1 Taking the Team Leader's Position

In the event of a suspected cardiac arrest it is critical that the team can perform various tasks at the same time, e.g. resuscitate the patient, coordinate and lead the team and collect the medical equipment (Husebø and Akerjordet 2016). In all briefings the facilitators demonstrated the team leader's spatial position. Since this had not been addressed previously the students did not understand where they should stand and why. To illustrate this, the facilitator used a wide range of instructional methods. First, the facilitator would regularly *demonstrate* where to stand by taking the right position herself and then show how this simultaneously enabled the team leader to ventilate the patient (manikin) and to lead the team. The space behind the head of the bed forms the basis for a central spatial position for executing the resuscitation algorithm in line with the guidelines. This position also enables a spatial overview for the team leader when ventilating the patient in cardiac arrest. It is critical that the nursing students understand where and how to position themselves since this location serves as an important prerequisite to carrying out specific actions and responsibilities connected to the position, both in clinical practice and in simulation. Second, the facilitator let the students *re-demonstrate* teamwork and individual skills. Third, the facilitators *make use of the students' displayed understandings* to further adjust their performance. In the excerpts presented below, it is demonstrated how such instructional problems are played out in close detail. Just before the situation occurs, the facilitator has demonstrated how to remove the headboards and pillows when ventilating the manikin. She has now positioned herself behind the head of the bed (Fig. 4.1).

By saying, "Do you see that when I stand here, I get a complete overview?" and simultaneously making a semicircle with her arms (Fig. 4.1, line 1–4), the facilitator demonstrates that this position is of importance and concerns the leader of the team. It is also associated with special responsibilities inasmuch as this person has a complete overview and leads the team. Moreover, there are certain expectations related to the position and team member, although these are not mentioned explicitly. The facilitator's arm gestures serve to frame and extend the spatial environment around the manikin's bed to be included in the "overview". By looking at the students and saying: "do you", the facilitator directly addresses her instruction to the student group. She also directly refers to her own position by saying, "when I stand here" (line 1). Using the deictic word "here" she shows and points out that her bodily position is spatially related to what is being said (Schegloff 1984). By employing a range of resources i.e. the body, gestures, gaze and verbal directives she points out a significant rule, "you have to stand here", thus making the spatial position central in the subsequent simulation scenario. Although the facilitator demonstrates exactly where and how to position herself, this does not mean that the whole student group is attentive and understands where to position themselves to lead the team and ventilate the patient.

The next excerpt (Fig. 4.1, Excerpt 2) illustrates *how the student displays* that she does not understand the instruction and how the facilitator *uses the student's exhibited understanding to correct* her performance of where to stand when ventilating

Excerpt 1

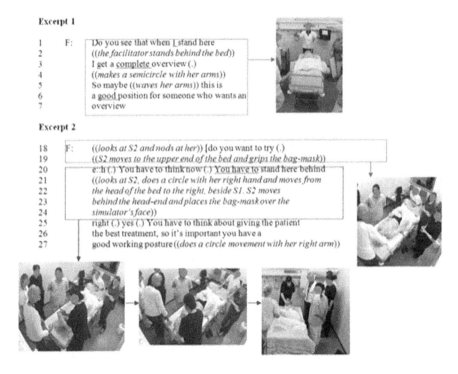

```
1    F:    Do you see that when I stand here
2          ((the facilitator stands behind the bed))
3          I get a complete overview (.)
4          ((makes a semicircle with her arms))
5          So maybe ((waves her arms)) this is
6          a good position for someone who wants an
7          overview
```

Excerpt 2

```
18   F:    ((looks at S2 and nods at her)) [do you want to try (.)
19         ((S2 moves to the upper end of the bed and grips the bag-mask))
20         e:h (.) You have to think now (.) You have to stand here behind
21         ((looks at S2, does a circle with her right hand and moves from
22         the head of the bed to the right, beside S1. S2 moves
23         behind the head-end and places the bag-mask over the
24         simulator's face))
25         right (.) yes (.) You have to think about giving the patient
26         the best treatment, so it's important you have a
27         good working posture ((does a circle movement with her right arm))
```

Fig. 4.1 Taking the team leader's position (Reproduced from Husebø et al. 2011)

the patient. A few minutes after the facilitator has given a brief demonstration of the bag-mask in the spatial position, she changes orientation to one of the students. By looking and nodding at S2 and simultaneously asking "do you want to try?" (line 18) the facilitator asks the student to *re-demonstrate* the bag-mask on the manikin. S2 responds by moving to the upper end of the bed and takes hold of the bag-mask from the side position (line 19). She places herself outside the spatial area the facilitator has indicated and still occupies. The facilitator sees that it is how and where S2 is standing (line 21) that could be a potential problem for ventilation and leadership. Where and how she stands are visible events which the facilitator can use as a resource for correcting the student's actions (Goodwin 1994). The facilitator responds by looking at S2, performing a circle movement with her right hand and moving her body to the left and out of the spatial environment (line 22) and simultaneously gives a directive, "you have to stand here, behind" (line 20). S2 responds to the facilitator's directive by moving to the previously demonstrated position behind the head of the bed. This bodily action, which provides her exhibited understanding, is visible evidence that the student has understood the facilitator's instructions (Sacks 1992, p. 252) and shows that verbal claims of understandings are not necessary in this case.

Although the facilitator demonstrated the spatial position in both resuscitation and simulation teams, a common instructional problem in all briefings was that the nursing students did not always understand how and where to stand and the reasons for this. The facilitators in monitoring the students' movements, regularly used the students' exhibited understanding to correct how and where they should stand to be able to both lead the team and ventilate the patient in the subsequent simulation scenario. Overall, this points to the fact that demonstrating the spatial position is necessary but not sufficient for the students to achieve a comprehensive understanding of its centrality to resuscitation teamwork. Further, re-demonstrations by the students effectively revealed potential (mis-) understandings and these re-demonstrations gave ample opportunities for the facilitators to both correct students' performance and elaborate reasons for why this specific position is critical in resuscitation.

4.2.3.2   Keeping Airways Open

Placing the oral airway in line with the guidelines is a prerequisite for opening airways in unconscious patients (Rumball and MacDonald 1997). Although trained in advance, a recurrent instructional problem was the students' difficulties in understanding how to apply the oral airway to the manikin. The students were able to answer the facilitator's questions concerning why and how the oral airway should be used, but in most groups, they were not able to *demonstrate* how to follow the guidelines for placing it. In turn, this was used by the facilitator to further *instruct* and *reinforce* important points for the whole student group. The second example illustrates how the student's verbal answer to the facilitator's question is insufficient in displaying relevant understanding, since the subsequent *demonstration* shows an inappropriate technique according to the guidelines. The sequence also shows a typical instance of how such deviances are also made use of for providing further instructions by the facilitator to the whole student group. In Fig. 4.2 the facilitator has just removed the headboard of the bed and positioned herself behind the bed.

She initiates a discussion by asking, "An oral airway – what's the purpose of it?" (line 32) as she simultaneously looks at the students and the five students look towards her. She changes her orientation by looking at S2, who has raised his hand (line 36). By responding with a "yes", the facilitator gives the go ahead to S2 to answer the question. S2's response, "so that the tongue shouldn't slide back in the throat", which displays a claimed understanding of the task. This is picked up and repeated by the facilitator as she asks S2, "would you like to place it?" (line 37–38). S2 responds by moving behind the head of the bed and rapidly putting the oral airway in the manikin's throat (line 39–40). This action requires a complex set of fine motor patterns and recognition of key spatial relationships between the oral airway and the oral cavity, and an understanding of the adjustments necessary to suit the physical conditions in the throat. S2 uses his fingers to push the oral airway in a straight, forward position into the manikin's throat, saying, "There, I believe" when he finishes the maneuver. It is how the student puts the oral airway in the "patient's" mouth that is of particular relevance here (line 39–40). In doing this, his *exhibited understanding* of placing the oral airway displays deviant performance, which is

Excerpt 3

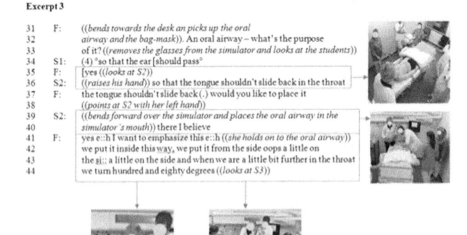

31	F:	((*bends towards the desk an picks up the oral*
32		*airway and the bag-mask*)). An oral airway – what's the purpose
33		of it? ((*removes the glasses from the simulator and looks at the students*))
34	S1:	(4) °so that the ear [should pass°
35	F:	[yes ((*looks at S2*))
36	S2:	((*raises his hand*)) so that the tongue shouldn't slide back in the throat
37	F:	the tongue shouldn't slide back (.) would you like to place it
38		((*points at S2 with her left hand*))
39	S2:	((*bends forward over the simulator and places the oral airway in the*
40		*simulator's mouth*)) there I believe
41	F:	yes e::h I want to emphasize this e::h ((*she holds on to the oral airway*))
42		we put it inside this way, we put it from the side oops a little on
43		the si:: a little on the side and when we are a little bit further in the throat
44		we turn hundred and eighty degrees ((*looks at S3*))

Fig. 4.2 Keeping airways open (Reproduced from Husebø et al. 2011)

immediately available to the facilitator and used as a basis for further corrections and explanation of the technique. The facilitator stands beside S2 and re-demonstrates the inserting of the oral airway in the manikin's mouth (line 43–44) as she verbally explains, "We put it in this way". The term "this way" in combination with gripping the oral airway upside down (line 42) underlines the right angle for inserting the oral airway to S2 and the whole student group. To further demonstrate the spatial point of rotating the oral airway in the throat, she grasps it with her fingers and says, "when we are a little bit further into the throat, we turn one hundred and eighty degrees" (line 43). In demonstrating execution of the oral airway, the facilitator draws on a wide range of resources: verbal explanation, body movements and gaze, hand and finger movements in relation to the material (the oral airway and the manikin) and how the oral airway relates to the anatomy of the throat. She refers to the patient in anatomical terms rather than simulation terms, thereby creating legitimacy for clinical practice (Johnson 2009). The facilitator (the expert) sees that the student puts the oral airway inside the mouth of the patient at an angle opposite to what it should be (see Goodwin's 1994 insightful analysis of "professional vision") (line 39–40) and uses the students' deviant performance, as displayed through his exhibited understanding, in *re-demonstrating* how to achieve open airways to the whole student group. Nevertheless, it cannot be taken for granted that S2 knows how perform the task in line with the guidelines either in the simulation or in clinical practice, since the angle S2 employed is not explicitly commented on and he is not encouraged to perform a second demonstration so that the facilitator is able to check if he could perform the task.

A recurrent instructional problem in the briefings on how to keep open airways was that a claimed understanding does not provide sufficient evidence of how to place oral airways in line with the instructions. Further, a student's demonstration often displays inaccurate understanding according to the instructions, which can be used for further re-demonstration directed to the whole student group. Finally, in re-demonstrations, facilitators typically refer to the artificial airways of the manikin in anatomical terms as if concerning a living patient, and thereby foreground the relevance of the task to real resuscitation teamwork.

To sum up, the analyses of both tasks reveal five critical aspects of preparing the students for the following scenario:

- The facilitator makes use of the simulation environment to *demonstrate* teamwork principles and individual tasks
- The facilitator let the students *re-demonstrate* teamwork and individual tasks
- A *claimed understanding* does not provide sufficient evidence of how to follow instructions.
- The facilitator uses the student's *exhibited understanding* to correct her/his performance
- Facilitators make use of students' inaccurate understanding for further re-demonstrations *directed to the whole student group*.

4.2.4   Discussion

The detailed and real-time investigation of briefings in simulated resuscitation teamwork in nursing education reveal features of instructional work that would otherwise remain hidden, for example, how the facilitator is attentive to the students' conduct in order to gauge their understanding. The facilitator's professional competence is not solely tied to the application of teamwork and individual skills, but also to the pedagogic concerns of monitoring the students to ensure that they have understood what they need for following the recommended guidelines in the subsequent scenario. It is worth returning to Sacks' (1992) distinction between "claiming" and "exhibiting" understanding regarding the pedagogical demonstration of the spatial position connected to the team leader role and its relevant responsibilities. The facilitator does not treat the student's speech in isolation from the student's displayed understandings as shown through their body language and actions. Accepting a claim as evidence of understanding may be sufficient when verifying, for example, that a student knows why a particular medical device is used, but it is not adequate for verifying that the student can execute specific tasks. The results reveal how facilitators seek evidence of understanding, not only through the students' verbal communication, but also through their observations of the students' practical actions

(Hindmarsh et al. 2014). The communicative resources for doing this include speech, gestures, gaze, a number of artefacts (the manikin, the bed, oral airway and bag-mask) and the physical environment (Goodwin 1994). The instructional work could not have been performed without the facilitators and students being able to perceive each other's actions in combination with verbal utterances. In other words, the facilitator and nursing students concertedly worked out, step by step, how to act with regards to appropriate resuscitation teamwork and the specific conditions of the simulation itself. Here, the facilitators' competence involves revealing potential problems by "reading" the students exhibited understandings. The facilitator sees that the student's spatial position (Fig. 4.1) and the angle of the oral airway (Fig. 4.2) would not be adequate if a cardiac arrest occurred. A kind of "Professional vision" (Goodwin 1994) is thus employed to detect and to instruct the student as well as the rest of the group. The spatial position is shown and made "accountable (observable-and-reportable) for all practical purposes" (Garfinkel 1967, p. vii).

Furthermore, this case, involving novices in the field, shows how briefings may involve a double instructional challenge for facilitators, i.e. both to ensure that the participants understand how to perform resuscitation and, at the same time, how this should be performed in the simulation. This means that the nursing students must learn both appropriate teamwork performance in relation to clinical practice and the specific conditions for how such actions should be carried out in relation to the simulation. The results point to the risk of disregarding the deviant conditions in the simulation, which might cause confusion and result in misconceptions (Chow and Naik 2008). This conclusion is supported by the studies of Escher et al. (2017), Johansson et al. (2017), Johnson (2007), and Rystedt and Lindwall (2004), who demonstrated how instructional work is critical for upholding the simulation as a relevant representation of clinical practice. The results highlight that the briefing is more than a general introduction to the activity, learning objectives, roles, simulation environment and medical equipment. It is also critical for creating a framework for understanding what the simulation is actually a simulation of (Hopwood et al. 2016).

4.2.5   Conclusions

The results of the study emphasize the tacit, often taken for granted aspects of instructions and points to the briefing as a much more complex and critical to the simulation scenario than presented in simulation textbooks and research in simulation.

- Firstly, the results point to how the instruction of novices might impose a double challenge in comparison to team training of professionals. It is, not only, necessary to understand how to adapt to the specific conditions of the simulation, but also to learn the mastery of a wide range of skills (often referred to as technical and non-technical respectively) and how these are to be simultaneously employed in coordinated teamwork.

- Secondly, that it is critical that briefings are arranged so that the students' exhibited understanding is available for facilitators to further their understandings of how to perform resuscitation teamwork. This implies an awareness of the differences between what students claim they understand and what they do as evidence for their understanding.
- Thirdly, it is essential that the facilitators' instructions are sensitive to these understandings to bridge between simulation and clinical practice and for achieving a shared understanding of what actually is going to be simulated.
- Finally, it is of crucial importance to learn from simulations is that facilitators' instructions explicate both relevant similarities and irrelevant differences between the simulation and resuscitation teamwork in real life settings.

Transcription Notes

The original video recordings were in Norwegian and have been translated to English by the first author. Students are marked as S1, S3 and S3 and facilitator as F. The episodes we present were transcribed using a notation inspired by Heath et al. (2010). Pauses are represented by numbers of seconds within brackets, with (.) indicating micro pauses, and concurrent talk horizontally aligned, with square brackets marking the onset of overlap. Extended vowel sounds are marked with colons, as in e::h. Enclosing a sequence in asterisks * indicates talk in a laughing tone. Underlining indicates stressed words, whereas the degree symbol ° means that the speech enclosed was noticeably quieter. Extra-linguistic action is included as comments within double parentheses, with italicized letters serving to better distinguish these from talk. Furthermore, the transcript is complemented with pictures that represent the gestures of the facilitator and students.

References

Arafeh, J. M. R., Hansen, S. S., Nichols, A. (2010). Debriefing in simulated-based learning: Facilitating a reflective discussion...[corrected] [published erratum appears in J PERINAT NEONAT NURS 2011 Jul/Sep; 25(3)268]. *Journal of Perinatal & Neonatal Nursing, 24*(4), 302–311. https://doi.org/10.1097/JPN.0b013e3181f6b5ec.

Bailey, C., Johnson-Russell, J., Lupien, A. (2010). High-fidelity patient simulation. In A. J. Lowenstein, & M. J. Bradshaw (Eds.), *Innovative teaching strategies in nursing and related health professions* (pp. 207–226). Sudbury: Jones and Bartlett Publishers.

Bartlett, J. L., Thomas-Wright, J., Pugh, H. (2014). When is it okay to cry? An end-of-life simulation experience. *Journal of Nursing Education, 53*(11), 659–662. https://doi.org/10.3928/01484834-20141023-02.

Beard, R. (2013). *Exploring the lived experiences of participants in simulation-based learning activities.* ProQuest LLC. Retrieved from http://search.ebscohost.com/login.aspx?direct=true&db=eric&AN=ED564615&scope=site

Bogossian, F., Cooper, S., Cant, R., Beauchamp, A., Porter, J., Kain, V., et al. (2014). Undergraduate nursing students' performance in recognising and responding to sudden patient deterioration in high psychological fidelity simulated environments: An Australian multi-centre study. *Nurse Education Today, 34*(5), 691–696. https://doi.org/10.1016/j.nedt.2013.09.015.

Calhoun, A. W., Boone, M. C., Porter, M. B., Miller, K. H. (2014). Using simulation to address hierarchy-related errors in medical practice. *Permanente Journal, 18*(2), 14–20. https://doi.org/10.7812/TPP/13-124.

Chow, R., & Naik, V. (2008). Realism and the art of simulation. In R. R. Kyle, & W. B. Murray (Eds.), *Clinical simulation: Operations, engineering, and management* (pp. 643–646). Amsterdam: Elsevier Academic.

Dieckmann, P. (2009). *Using simulations for education, training and research.* Lengerich: Pabst.

Escher, C., Rystedt, H., Creutzfeldt, J., Meurling, L., Nystrom, S., Dahlberg, J., et al. (2017). Method matters: Impact of in-scenario instruction on simulation-based teamwork training. *Advances in Simulation, 2*(25). https://doi.org/10.1186/s41077-017-0059-9.

Garfinkel, H. (1967). *Studies in ethnomethodology.* Englewood Cliffs: Prentice-Hall.

Goodwin, C. (1994). Professional vision. *American Anthropologist, 96*(3), 606–633. https://doi.org/10.1525/aa.1994.96.3.02a00100.

Have, P. T. (2007). *Doing conversation analysis: A practical guide* (2nd edn). London: Sage.

Heath, C., & Hindmarsh, J. (2002). Analysing interaction: Video, ethnography and situated conduct. In T. May (Ed.), *Qualitative research in action* (pp. 99–121). London: SAGE.

Heath, C., Hindmarsh, J., Luff, P. (2010). *Video in qualitative research. Analysing social interaction in everyday life* (Vol. 1). Los Angeles: SAGE.

Hindmarsh, J., Hyland, L., Banerjee, A. (2014). Work to make simulation work: 'Realism', instructional correction and the body in training. *Discourse Studies, 16*(2), 247–269. https://doi.org/10.1177/1461445613514670.

Hopwood, N., Rooney, D., Boud, D., Kelly, M. (2016). Simulation in higher education: A sociomaterial view. *Educational Philosophy and Theory, 48*(2), 165–178.

Husebø, S. E. (2012). *Conditions for learning in simulation practice: Training for team-based resuscitation in nursing education.* (no. 173). Stavanger: University of Stavanger, Faculty of Social Sciences, Department of Health Studies.

Husebø, S. E., & Akerjordet, K. (2016). Quantitative systematic review of multi-professional teamwork and leadership training to optimize patient outcomes in acute hospital settings. *Journal of Advanced Nursing, 72*(12), 2980–3000. 10.1111/jan.13035.

Husebø, S. E., Friberg, F., Søreide, E., Rystedt, H. (2012). Instructional problems in briefings: How to prepare nursing students for simulation-based cardiopulmonary resuscitation training. *Clinical Simulation in Nursing, 8*(7), e307–e318. https://doi.org/10.1016/j.ecns.2010.12.002.

Husebø, S. E., Rystedt, H., Friberg, F. (2011). Educating for teamwork – nursing students' coordination in simulated cardiac arrest situations. *Journal of Advanced Nursing, 67*(10), 2239–2255. https://doi.org/10.1111/j.1365-2648.2011.05629.x.

INACSL. (2016a). INACSL standards of best practice: Simulation facilitation. *Clinical Simulation in Nursing, 12*, 16–20. https://doi.org/10.1016/j.ecns.2016.09.007.

INACSL. (2016b). INACSL standards of best practice: Simulation simulation glossary. *Clinical Simulation in Nursing, 12*, 39–47. https://doi.org/10.1016/j.ecns.2016.09.012.

Johansson, E., Lindwall, O., Rystedt, H. (2017). Experiences, appearances, and interprofessional training: The instructional use of video in post-simulation debriefings. *International Journal of Computer-Supported Collaborative Learning, 12*(1), 91–112. https://doi.org/10.1007/s11412-017-9252-z.

Johnson, E. (2007). Surgical simulators and simulated surgeons: Reconstituting medical practice and practitioners in simulations. *Social Studies of Science, 37*(4), 585–608.

Johnson, E. (2009). Extending the simulator: Good practice for instructors using medical simulators. In P. Dieckmann (Ed.), *Using simulations for education, training and research* (pp. 180–201). Berlin: Pabst Science Publisher.

Kelly, M. A., Hager, P., Gallagher, R. (2014). What matters most? Students' rankings of simulation components that contribute to clinical judgment. *Journal of Nursing Education, 53*(2), 97–101. https://doi.org/10.3928/01484834-20140122-08.

Kolbe, M., Grande, B., Spahn, D. R. (2015). Briefing and debriefing during simulation-based training and beyond: Content, structure, attitude and setting. *Best Practice & Research. Clinical Anaesthesiology, 29*(1), 87–96. https://doi.org/10.1016/j.bpa.2015.01.002.

Koo, L., Layson-Wolf, C., Brandt, N., Hammersla, M., Idzik, S., Rocafort, P. T., et al. (2014). Qualitative evaluation of a standardized patient clinical simulation for nurse practitioner and pharmacy students. *Nurse Education in Practice, 14*(6), 740–746. https://doi.org/10.1016/j.nepr.2014.10.005.

Lopreiato, J. O., Downing, D., Gammon, W., Lioce, L., Sittner, B. J., Slot, V., et al. (2016). Healthcare simulation dictionary. Retrieved from http://www.ssih.org/dictionary

Morrison, A. M., & Catanzaro, A. M. (2010). High-fidelity simulation and emergency preparedness. *Public Health Nursing, 27*(2), 164–173. https://doi.org/10.1111/j.1525.1446.2010.00838.x.

Nestel, D., & Gough, S. (2018). Designing simulation-based learning activities: A systematic approach. In D. Nestel, M. Kelly, B. Jolly, M. Watson (Eds.), *Healthcare simulation education: Evidence, theory & practice* (pp. 135–142). Wiley.

Nestel, D., Kelly, M., Jolly, B., Watson, M. (2018). *Healthcare simulation education: Evidence, theory & practice*. Wiley.

NNR. (2015). Guidelines for resuscitation. Retrieved from http://nrr.org/images/pdf/HLR_med_hjertestarter_Norske_retningslinjer_2015.pdf

Rudolph, J. W., Raemer, D. B., Simon, R. (2014). Establishing a safe container for learning in simulation: The role of the presimulation briefing. *Simulation in Healthcare, 9*(6), 339–349. https://doi.org/10.1097/sih.0000000000000047.

Rumball, C. J., & MacDonald, D. (1997). The PTL, combitube, laryngeal mask, and oral airway: A randomized prehospital comparative study of ventilatory device effectiveness and cost-effectiveness in 470 cases of cardiorespiratory arrest. *Prehospital Emergency Care, 1*(1), 1–10.

Rystedt, H., & Lindwall, O. (2004). The interactive construction of learning foci in simulation-based learning environments: A case study of an anaesthesia course. *PsychNology Journal, 2*(2), 168–188.

Rystedt, H., & Sjöblom, B. (2012). Realism, authenticity, and learning in healthcare simulations: Rules of relevance and irrelevance as interactive achievements. *Instructional Science, 40*(5), 785–789. https://doi.org/10.1007/s11251-012-9213-x.

Sacks, H., Jefferson, G., Schegloff, E. A. (1992). *Lectures on conversation: 2* (Vol. 2). Oxford: Blackwell.

Schegloff, E. A. (1984). On some gestures' relation to talk. In J. Atkinson, & J. Heritage (Eds.), *Studies in conversation analysis* (pp. 266–296). Cambridge, UK: Cambridge University Press.

4.3 Facilitators In-Scenario Challenges in Inter-Professional Simulation-Based Team Training of Non-technical Skills

Cecilia Escher · Johan Creutzfeldt · Lisbet Meurling · Li Felländer-Tsai
Karolinska Institutet
Stockholm, Sweden
email: cecilia.escher@ki.se; johan.creutzfeldt@ki.se
lisbet.meurling@ki.se; li.tsai@ki.se

4.3.1 Introduction

In this section, we focus on and discuss important aspects for educators to consider when connecting the simulated scenario to a desired learning outcome. In line with principles of constructive alignment (Biggs and Tang 2007) a scenario should enable practice of the pre-defined, intended learning outcomes. Working to create a constructive alignment in teaching makes it necessary for the educator to clarify the learning objectives and guide the activities accordingly throughout the simulation.

Our example focuses on Inter-professional Simulation-based Teamwork Training (SBTT) that has non-technical skills as learning objectives. Non-technical skills can be described as the cognitive, social and personal resource skills that complement technical skills, and contribute to safe and efficient task performance (Flin 2008). Crew resource management (CRM) can be described as the effective use of all available resources for flight crew personnel to assure a safe and efficient operation, reducing error, avoiding stress and increasing efficiency (Helmreich et al. 1999), and is a commonly used approach to the training of non-technical skills also in health care settings.

We claim that the educator needs to consider that a simulation is valuable only if learning can be transferred from the simulated setting into clinical practice. We draw on empirical research and extensive experience in order to discuss three important aspects of the educator's tasks in simulation-based learning; Firstly, we will illustrate specific challenges when introducing and conducting interprofessional simulations with non-technical skills as learning objectives by using a previously described program for non-technical skills. Secondly, we will discuss scenario realism and the fidelity concept (authenticity) from an educator's and learners' perspectives.

Thirdly, we will describe methods used by facilitators to bridge the gap to reality during simulated scenarios. Based on empirical research, the impact of practice on participants' actions are illuminated. In summary, this section will provide guidance for educators in inter-professional SBTT with non-technical skills learning objectives. The alignment of scenarios and assessment as well as the complex task of in-scenario instruction will be specifically addressed.

4.3.1.1 The Educator in Simulation-Based Team Training

The interprofessional learning activity in simulation-based teamwork training is quite different from other medical education learning tasks in more traditional settings. Participants as well as educators point at the familiarity with the concept of SBTT is needed in order to lead successful sessions (Parsh 2010; Harder et al. 2013). Familiarity with the SBTT concept is regarded as necessary to reach a rich understanding based on both experience, reflection and abstraction.

A number of roles and skills are required from the educator, in order be able to deliver simulation-based education of high quality. To describe the role of an educator in this area, Harden and Crosby published a guide outlining the 12 roles of a medical teacher (Harden and Crosby 2000). Six roles of relevance for simulation-based education were summarized as:

1. Information provider
2. Role model
3. Facilitator
4. Assessor
5. Planner
6. Resource developer

These roles are applied during different phases of a simulation session (Dieckmann 2007; Dieckmann et al. 2009; Harden and Crosby 2000). In simulation literature *facilitator* is a term used for faculty engaged in simulation-based teamwork training, most commonly for instruction during and after scenarios. Work by Johnson (2007) underscores how simulations can be meaningful learning experiences if facilitators help participants by adding information from clinical work. She also points at the importance of the facilitator as role model, especially for junior learners.

4.3.1.2   Specific Challenges When Introducing Inter-professional Simulations with Non-technical Skills as Learning Objectives

The term *non-technical skills* (Sect. 4.3.2) and the related *crew resource management* concept (Sect. 4.3.4) is derived from industries such as aviation (Flin 2008) and has been adopted to healthcare. Although many bodies including the WHO (2009) have embraced the importance of non-technical skills the concept is not yet universally known in all healthcare organizations, therefore teamwork skills can host different interpretations. As healthcare organizations commonly have not established a gold standard for, or common definition of, teamwork skills, students' and professionals' perceptions and level of knowledge has been shown to be diverse (Flin 2008). The uncertainty regarding gold standard in regard to non-technical skills may be due to the fact that these skills differ distinctly as compared to algorithm-based treatments such as cardiopulmonary resuscitation where guidelines are standardized, upgraded regularly and accepted by all professional organizations. This uncertainty poses challenges to facilitators when introducing and facilitating simulations.

4.3.2   The Crew Resource Management (CRM) Concept

In Sect. 7.2 the historical roots of simulation-based education are traced to other areas than education, such as the military and aviation domains. The CRM concept for the training of non-technical skills was launched in aviation in the 1980s as a response to several accidents (Helmreich et al. 1999) in order to improve task performance for frontline staff. The concept has been continuously developed, and regular simulation-based team training founded on CRM principles is now since many years a routine in civil aviation. The overarching aim of CRM is to identify and use all available resources in terms of information, equipment and people (Helmreich et al. 1999; Pierre 2011) in emergency situations.

Training courses in CRM have been developed for many industries, including aviation, offshore, shipping, railways. Training courses have also been adjusted to and accepted in healthcare settings (Gaba et al. 1991). Some of the differences between aviation and healthcare teams are that emergency teams in healthcare are often larger and more dynamic in terms of team members as compared to teams in aviation. Nonetheless, principles from CRM have been found very helpful in health-care settings (Chassin and Galvin 1998; Gaba et al. 2001; Flin and Maran 2015). The principles represent a variety of skills and tools for better interaction and safe and predictable performance in routine as well as under emergency conditions. CRM training for safe performance in healthcare was first adopted in anesthesia (Chassin and Galvin 1998; Gaba et al. 2001) and training modules based on "aviation-style" CRM for anesthesiologists started in the end of the 1980s. Since then, the importance of non-technical skills for safe healthcare has been acknowledged worldwide. The applicability of non-technical skills gained acceptance in a wide range of health-care settings during the 1990:ies and is now taught and trained at undergraduate as well as postgraduate levels in many acute care settings (Pierre 2011). Healthcare CRM is commonly taught in simulation-based and classroom-based team training courses. There are several classroom-based teaching concepts that have been shown to improve patient safety (Kemper et al. 2016; Arora et al. 2012; Morey et al. 2002; Neily et al. 2010). CRM in health care has also been shown to increase the return of investment by lowering frequencies of adverse events (Moffat-Bruce et al. 2017). E-learning and serious games have also been used successfully for non-technical skills teaching (Creutzfeldt et al. 2012; Gaupp et al. 2016).

4.3.2.1 CRM in Simulation-Based Teamwork Training (SBTT)

In healthcare, the CRM concept is a common foundation for simulation-based teamwork training with clinicians. The training model is supported by findings of positive correlations to patient safety (Østergaard et al. 2011). Studies display positive effects of SBTT on learning (O'Dea et al. 2014; Oxelmark et al. 2017), particularly regarding knowledge of teamwork tools, perception of abilities to perform efficiently in emergency situations and on staff's attitudes (Arora et al. 2015; Ruesseler et al. 2012; Meurling et al. 2013), e.g. towards creating a patient safety climate. Transfer of learning from SBTT has also been found to improve patient safety (Patterson et al. 2013; Draycott et al. 2006; Capella et al. 2010).

In order to assess and train team skills/non-technical skills in clinical settings and in SBTT, a number of profession-specific behavior rating scales have been developed. Some examples are Anaesthetists' Non-Technical Skills (Fletcher et al. 2003). Non-Technical Skills for Surgeons (Yule et al. 2008) and Scrub Practitioners List of Non-Technical Skills (Mitchell et al. 2013). Rating scales to guide assessment and training of non-technical skills in a clinical environment have been developed to form a gold standard for teamwork for professional clinicians and enable goal directed training. When viewing the implications for educators providing crew resource management training it becomes evident that there is a need to identify and anchor successful key behaviors that are in alignment with the training goals, and that can guide the debriefing and assessment of the training.

To enable the facilitator to use one common tool for all professions in this endeavor, a program for assessment of All Team Members non-technical skills (ATEAM) was developed at the Center for Advanced Medical Simulation and

Training (CAMST.) The program was published in 2009 (Wallin et al. 2009). ATEAM includes team leaders' as well as followers' behaviour. It can be used in different clinical settings and is therefore particularly helpful in inter-professional settings. In the following we provide a theoretical description of the program and how facilitators can apply this in the SBTT.

4.3.2.2 Anchoring and Assessing Behavior and Learning Goals in SBTT: The ATEAM Program

The constructive alignment concept for successful learning activities highlights the necessity of harmonizing educational objectives, working forms and assessment on the goals to achieve the intended outcome of activities (Biggs and Tang 2007). If a simulation has non-technical learning goals, scenarios needs to address for example effective communication in an appropriate context (that is adjusted to the participants). In order to introduce and facilitate inter-professional SBTT a framework, gold standard, for anchoring and assessing team behaviors is necessary.

The main non-technical skills categories of the ATEAM program that identify, and anchor participants' successful key behaviors are to what extent he or she:

1. Takes a team member role, with the subcategories – all team members' behavior, leader behavior and follower behavior
2. Gathers information and communicates
3. Contributes to a shared understanding of the situation
4. Makes collaborative decisions
5. Coordinates and executes tasks

Each category, and subset, has verbal anchors at four levels, *Poor, In need of improvement, Good* and *Proficient*. A common understanding of the training goals is the foundation of SBTT and enables facilitators and participants to meet on common ground in the assessment. Non-technical skills such as "a shared understanding of the situation" and "makes collaborative decisions" are not easily explained to clinicians or students without prior knowledge. The verbal anchors of the program facilitate clarification of key behaviors and can be used in various educational activities around simulation, such as discussions, seminars, in simulations and as a preparation before SBTT. Facilitators in SBTT can use the program to ensure equality regarding assessment and guidance in debriefing after scenarios. The program has also been used for assessment of resident physicians in clinical teamwork situations (Fig. 4.3).

4.3.3 Scenario Fidelity and Realism (Authenticity) in SBTT

Facilitators have to consider several aspects of special importance for participants' learning during SBTT and subsequent transfer to real-world settings. In order to benefit from the simulation scenario as an experiential learning situation, i.e.

Fig. 4.3 The ATEAM program (Wallin et al. 2009)

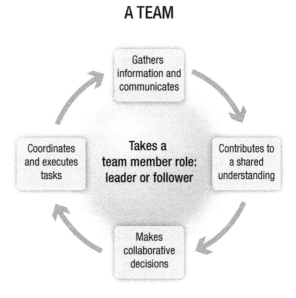

learning by reflection on experience (Dieckmann 2007; Kolb 1984; Rystedt and Sjöblom 2012) facilitators and also participants have to buy into the concept. It is considered to be important to act "as-if" (Dieckmann 2007) the simulation was a real situation i.e. enabling immersion. Therefore, simulated scenarios have to make sense to participants and manikins and equipment has to be "real enough" (Robinson and Mania 2007; Salas and Burke 2002) to match key attributes of the clinical case being simulated. The fidelity concept is used to describe resemblance of a simulation to the real world. Many publications address the fidelity concept e.g. Paige and Morin (2013) who propose a matrix to conceptualize three dimensions of fidelity; physical, psychological and conceptual fidelity. Clapper et al. (2015) point to that the literature is not uniform in the use of the fidelity concept. Nestel et al. (2018) suggest adding a meaningfulness perspective to fidelity when describing simulation activities. A simulation can be meaningful without being realistic, for example well-made screen-based simulations. Simulations with high realism (structural fidelity) do not necessarily apply meaningfulness if the simulation is not adjusted to the participants in terms of level of difficulty or type of clinical case. Increasing the number of professions involved in interprofessional training, poses challenges to design scenarios that allow each member of staff to have purposeful tasks to perform to promote a high level of engagement (Creutzfeldt et al. 2016). It is to our experience also necessary to include representatives for all professional groups in the facilitator team to ensure practical relevance for all participants.

In recent years the traditional fidelity concept has been challenged (Norman et al. 2012). In an interview study on fiction and realism it was found that participants in simulations have diverse opinions regarding features that enhance reality (Dieckmann et al. 2007). It has been argued that the fidelity concept should be abandoned since several studies have failed to find a strong correlation between simulator fidelity and the perceived value of the simulation-based education and transfer of learning (Norman et al. 2012). To replace the fidelity concept Hamstra et al. (2014) suggest "functional task alignment". This construct emphasizes the realism of the simulation relative to the setting it is mimicking and the learning objectives. From our studies, we would also argue that the most important aspect contributing to the perceived realism of a simulation besides the material setting and the scenario, is the ways in-scenario instructions are delivered (Escher et al. 2017).

4.3.3.1 Aspects of SBTT Fidelity from the Facilitators' and Participants' View

Few studies have so far focused on facilitators' reactions in relation to different levels of simulation fidelities. A study by Meurling et al. (2014) compared how the level of manikin fidelity affected facilitators. Results displayed that using a low fidelity manikin was associated with higher mental strain among facilitators compared to using a higher fidelity manikin. This difference in mental strain was interesting as the participants in the study displayed a very different pattern with similar levels of mental strain using the two manikin fidelities. A possible mechanism for the small differences regarding participants' reactions when training with a lower or higher fidelity manikin could be facilitators' actions. By skillfully adding missing information facilitators seem to be able to compensate for the shortcomings of the simulator.

Lower fidelity simulators display fewer of the essential signs necessary for assessment and treatment, such as oxygen saturation and skin color, and in-scenario instruction is therefore more demanding for facilitators but not necessarily of less value for the participants. Rystedt and Sjöblom (2012) argue that the perceived fidelity is created in the interaction between participants, simulator and facilitators. By relating to real life experiences facilitators' play an important role to create valuable learning opportunities (Johnson 2007). These results are in the same vein as the ongoing discussion questioning the importance of simulator fidelity for learning (Norman et al. 2012; Dieckmann et al. 2007).

In an aforementioned study, facilitators found training using a low fidelity manikin as more demanding compared to a higher fidelity simulator, the possible explanation being that more information has to be conveyed by facilitators when using lower fidelity. Higher fidelity can, on the other hand be more demanding for facilitators depending on opportunities for technical support and the individual facilitator's confidence in using sophisticated technology (Harder et al. 2013). Facilitators' tasks are often not restricted to management of the simulator but also include management of video equipment, briefings, in-scenario instruction and debriefing. To enable high quality inter-professional SBTT more than one facilitator and technical expertise is necessary to run each scenario.

Considering participants' perception of realism in simulated scenarios a study by Dieckmann et al. (2007) revealed individual non-consistent perceptions of cues of reality and fiction. The participating anesthetists in Dieckmann's work took part in scenarios together with facilitators role-playing the other members of the operating room team. The anesthetists in the study perceived the same features as a reality cue in one and fiction in another scenario. Dieckmann and colleagues concluded that perception of realism relies on several features, one being the role-play by facilitators, another the opportunity to get clarification and ask questions during scenarios. Recent sociomaterial perspectives on SBTT, covered in depth in Sect. 2.2, in this volume, point at the interactive aspects of simulated scenarios including interactions between participants, facilitators, equipment and simulators (Nyström et al. 2016).

4.3.4 In-Scenario Facilitation to Fill the Gaps in SBTT

As all simulated settings will differ from clinical situations; participants will require assistance during scenarios in order to understand what is being simulated in order to fulfill learning goals. From the learners' perspective there is a skill to the simulation-based education itself, i.e. participants who take part in SBTT in a particular setting at a regular basis will "learn how to simulate". The regular participant will know what to expect in terms of assessment of the manikin and communication with facilitators during scenarios. Participants taking part for the first time in a particular clinical setting will require more assistance during scenarios compared to students and staff used to SBTT. There are several aspects to consider regarding in-scenario instruction that will be discussed in the following sections.

4.3.4.1 Help to Find and Use Equipment in SBTT

To optimize learning and focus on learning objectives it is often desirable to provide participants assistance regarding tasks that are not included in the learning objectives. This may include finding equipment and obtaining information regarding the setting, i.e. how to get in touch with other caregivers and results of investigations such as laboratory and radiology. Often the simulation uses equipment not perfectly matched to the clinical setting. Non-realistic equipment does not have to be a major disadvantage given the facilitators ability to bridge the difficulties and ensure that participants are not stuck with unknown equipment missing the learning opportunities of a scenario.

4.3.4.2 Feed-Back and Coaching in SBTT

There are educators who consider in-scenario feedback as particularly helpful for learning which is supported by research on deliberate practice by Ericsson (2008). Many educators agree that faculty should not accept too large deviations from the training goals as acting out the "wrong behavior" is unwanted. In aviation simulations, planes rarely crash since such an event can have a very negative impact on learners. Many healthcare educators agree that correspondingly patients should not die during SBTT unless breaking bad news is a learning objective (Heller et al. 2016).

There are several options to "save a scenario" (Dieckmann et al. 2010) if learning opportunities are at stake. One is to stop, debrief and restart the scenario, another is coaching by facilitators i.e. giving advice, adding information or asking a clarifying question. Simulations can benefit from facilitators' coaching for example algorithms and decision-making processes by clues and questions rather than leaving the participants to make a lot of mistakes and fail to treat the simulated patient. On the other hand, depending on the learning goals of the session and the possibilities to repeat the scenario, allowing participants to make mistakes can provide important experiential learning opportunities.

4.3.4.3   Providing Extra Scenario Information in SBTT

Facilitators in healthcare simulations must bridge the gap between the appearance of a patient simulator and the body of a sick patient. Human patient simulators can be highly sophisticated with features such as pupils that react to light, breathing sounds and exhaled carbon dioxide. However, some features are still very different from the body of a sick patient such as skin color and temperature, bodily movements and abdominal examination. This gap in bodily appearance must be filled out by facilitators to enable assessment and decision-making by participants. The necessary amount of supplementary information depends on the fidelity of the simulator and the scenario that it is mimicking.

The notion extra scenario information has been suggested to describe this sub-set of in-scenario instruction (Escher et al. 2017). In a study including video filmed scenarios from three Swedish simulation centers, four methods for extra scenario information were found in the dataset. The methods were:

1. A facilitator present in the simulation suite acting as a confederate.
2. A facilitator providing information from a bystander position.
3. Facilitators providing information from an adjacent room to participants via a speaker.
4. Facilitators providing information from an adjacent room to one of the participants via an earpiece.

Table 4.1 displays data from the study in relation to the research questions: what triggers facilitators to convey extra scenario information and what visible effect the method has on subsequent actions during the scenario. The study revealed that timing of information was essential for how scenarios played out. When teams were looking for important information such as bodily movements of the patient, they could not continue the assessment until they received that information. Further, team communication was impaired when participants kept asking for information or facilitators used a lot of time describing findings thereby hampering team communication. Facilitators situated closer to the action i.e. in the suite were superior regarding timing and extra scenario information was therefore less disturbing to participants' teamwork.

Table 4.1 Examples of methods for and impact of extra scenario information

Instruction	Trigger to get information	Visible impact on team activities
1. Facilitator as a part of the team, a confederate	Participants' actions and questions triggered prompt response from the facilitator. Gestures and position in the room were important resources	Immediate response. Shortcuts and scaffolding through questions and cues. Information on findings to everybody. Participants focused on the problem
2. Facilitator as a bystander in the simulator suite	Participants' actions and questions triggered prompt response from the facilitator standing close to the team	Immediate response. Speedy talk and coded information speeded up the work. Information on findings to everybody. Participants focused on the problem
3. Information from a facilitator outside the simulator room through a speaker	Leader telling what he was assessing triggered information from the facilitator. Sometimes delay in delivery of information	Lack of timing and lengthy messages was at times disruptive for the teamwork. Information on findings to everybody. At times communication was vertical towards the facilitator
4. Information from a facilitator outside the simulator room to one participant through an earpiece	Participants' actions and questions triggered response from the facilitator. Sometimes delay in delivery of information	Timing of information had an impact on the pace of work. Information to one participant had to be conveyed to the team. Participant with earpiece missed team communication when receiving information

Escher et al. (2017) conclude that there are several methods for extra scenario information. Methods used have substantial and diverse impact on scenarios and should be accustomed to training goals of a simulation.

The method used for extra scenario information is commonly not explicit in studies on SBTT and the knowledge base regarding in-scenario instruction is therefore scarce (Cheng et al. 2016). Prior studies are limited to the use of facilitators participating in scenarios (so called confederates), the use of bystander, earpiece and speaker has so far rarely been discussed. The slower response of the in-scenario instructions delivered by earpiece and loudspeaker can be beneficial for the learning in novice interprofessional teams but disruptive to professionals. In the literature the tasks carried out by a confederate varies considerably. Besides adding information and coaching, the use of a confederate offers opportunities for acting out for example difficult behavior of a team member and tuning the level of stress in the scenario. Nestel et al. (2014) concludes that successful use of a confederate in simulations demands scripted roles and educators with some acting skills. The use of confederates widens the applicability of SBTT as scenarios can be standardized and include a broader set of learning objectives such as speaking up to a team member and informing a relative. A facilitator in the role of a confederate can also fulfill other tasks during scenarios i.e. help to find equipment, feedback and coaching. Escher's et al. study (2017) shows that the facilitator as a confederate actor also has an impact on the problem focus and immediate response of the team.

4.3.5   Conclusions

• Simulation-based training puts special educational demands when focusing on non-technical skills in inter-professional teams. A program clarifying educational goals can guide educators to align training and assessment.
• When constructing scenarios, the facilitator needs to consider the perception of realism (authenticity) since it influences learning. Realism is influenced by fidelity of the simulator, but lower fidelity may be compensated for by in-scenario instructions and the material settings.
• During simulation-based teamwork training the facilitator needs to provide extra-scenario information to fill out reality gaps during the simulation. This can be carried out in several ways, but by having a confederate within the simulation, learning conditions can be adjusted and augmented.

References

Arora, S., Sevdalis, N., Ahmed, M. (2012). Safety skills training for surgeons: A half-day intervention improves knowledge, attitudes and awareness of patient safety. *Surgery, 152*(1), 26–31. https://doi.org/10.1016/j.surg.2012.02.006. [Published Online First: 2012/04/17].

Arora, S., Hull, L., Fitzpatrick, M. (2015). Crisis management on surgical wards: A simulation-based approach to enhancing technical, teamwork, and patient interaction skills. *Annals of Surgery.* https://doi.org/10.1097/sla.0000000000000824. [Published Online First: 2015/02/04].

Biggs, J., & Tang, C. (2007). *Teaching for quality learning at university* (3rd edn). New York: SRHE and open University Press.

Capella, J., Smith, S., Philp, A. (2010). Teamwork training improves the clinical care of trauma patients. *Journal of Surgical Education, 67*(6), 439–443. https://doi.org/10.1016/j.jsurg.2010.06.006.

Chassin, M. R., & Galvin, R. W. (2018). The urgent need to improve health care quality. Institute of Medicine National Roundtable on Health Care Quality. *JAMA, 1998*(280). https://doi.org/10.1001/jama.280.11.1000.

Cheng, A., Kessler, D., Mackinnon, R., Chang, T. P., Nadkarni, V. M., Hunt, E. A., et al. (2016). Reporting guidelines for health care simulation research extensions to the CONSORT and STROBE Statements. *Simulation in Healthcare, 11,* 238–248.

Clapper, T. C., Cornell, I. G., Tun, J. K. (2015). Redefining simulation fidelity for healthcare education. *Simulation and Gaming. 46*(2), 159–174. https://doi.org/10.1177/1046878115576103.

Creutzfeldt, J., Hedman, L., Felländer-Tsai, L. (2012). Effects of pre-training using serious game technology on CPR performance – an exploratory quasi-experimental transfer study. *Scandinavian Journal of Trauma, Resuscitation and Emergency Medicine,* (20), 79.

Creutzfeldt, J., Hedman, L., Felländer-Tsai, L. (2016). Cardiopulmonary resuscitation training by avatars: A qualitative study of medical students' experiences using a multiplayer virtual world. *JMIR Serious Games, 4*(2).

Dieckmann, R. (2007). Becoming a simulator instructor and learning to facilitate. In R. M. Kyle, & W. Bosseau (Eds.). *Clinical simulation: Operations, engineering and management.* Burlington: Academic. ProQuest ebrary. Web. 20 October 2015: Academic press 2007.

Dieckmann, P. (2007). Deepening the theoretical foundations of patient simulation as social practice. *Simulation in Healthcare, 2*(3), 183–193. https://doi.org/10.1097/SIH.0b013e3180f637f5.

Dieckmann, P., Molin Friis, S., Lippert, A., Østergaard, D. (2009). The art and science of debriefing in simulation: Ideal and practice. *Medical Teacher, 31*(7), e287–e294. https://doi.org/10.1080/01421590902866218.

Dieckmann P., Lippert, A., Glavin, R., Rall, M. (2010). When things do not go as expected: Scenario life savers. *Simulation in Healthcare, 5*(4), 219–225. https://doi.org/10.1097/SIH.0b013e3181e77f74.

Dieckmann, P., Manser, T., Wehner, T., Rall, M. (2007). Reality and fiction cues in medical patient simulation: An interview study with anesthesiologists. *Journal of Cognitive Engineering and Decision Making,1*(2), 148–168. https://doi.org/10.1518/155534307x232820.

Draycott, T., Sibanda, T., Owen L. (2006). Does training in obstetric emergencies improve neonatal outcome? *BJOG, 113*(2),177–182. https://doi.org/10.1111/j.1471-0528.2006.00800.x. [Published Online First: 2006/01/18].

Ericsson, K. A. (2008). Deliberate practice and acquisition of expert performance: A general overview. *Academic Emergency Medicine, 15*(11), 988–994. 10.1111/j.1553-2712.2008.00227.x.

Escher, C., Rystedt, H., Creutzfeldt, J., Meurling, L., Nyström, S., Dahlberg, J., et al. (2017). Method matters: Impact of in-scenario instruction on simulation-based teamwork training. *Advances in Simulation, 2*(25). https://doi.org/10.1186/s41077-017-0059-9.

Fletcher, G., Flin, R., McGeorge, P., Glavin, R., Maran, N., Patey, R. (2003). Anaesthetists' non-technical skills (ANTS): Evaluation of a behavioral marker system. *British Journal of Anaesthesia, 90*(5), 580–588. https://doi.org/10.1093/bja/aeg112.

Flin, R. H. (2008). *Safety at the sharp end: A guide to non-technical skills.* Aldershot: Ashgate.

Flin, R., & Maran, N. (2015). Basic concepts for crew resource management and non-technical skills. *Best Practice & Research Clinical Anaesthesiology, 29*(1), 27–39. https://doi.org/10.1016/j.bpa.2015.02.002.

Gaba, D. M., Howard, S. K., Fish, K. J., Yang, G., Samquist, F. H. (1991). Anesthesia crisis resource management training. *Anesthesiology, 75*(Supplement), A1062. 10.1097/00000542-199109001-01061.

Gaba, D. M., Howard, S. K., Fish, K. (2001). Simulation-based training in anesthesia crisis resource management (ACRM): A decade of experience. *Simulation & Gaming, 32*(2), 175.

Gaupp, R., Körner, M., Fabry, G. (2016). Effects of a case-based interactive e-learning course on knowledge and attitudes about patient safety: A quasi-experimental study with third-year medical students. *BMC Medical Education, 16*(1), 1–8. https://doi.org/10.1186/s12909-016-0691-4.

Harder, B. N., Ross, C. J. M., Paul, P. (2013). Instructor comfort level in high-fidelity simulation. *Nurse Education Today, 33*(10), 1242–1245. https://doi.org/10.1016/j.nedt.2012.09.003.

Harden, R. M., & Crosby, J. (2000). AMEE Guide No. 20: The good teacher is more than a lecturer – the twelve roles of the teacher. *Medical Teacher, 22*(4), 334–347.

Hamstra, S. J., Brydges, R., Hatala, R., Zendejas, B., Cook, D. A. (2014). Reconsidering fidelity in simulation-based training. *Academic Medicine, 89*(3), 387–392.

Heller, J. B., Demaria, A. S., Katz T. D., Heller, J. A., Goldberg, A. T. (2016). Death during simulation: A literature review. *Journal of Continuing Education in the Health Professions, 36*(4), 316–322. https://doi.org/10.1097/CEH.0000000000000116.

Helmreich, R. L., Merritt, A. C., Wilhelm, J. A. (1999). The evolution of crew resource management training in commercial aviation. *The International Journal of Aviation Psychology, 9*(1), 19–32. https://doi.org/10.1207/s15327108ijap0901_2.

Johnson, E. (2007). Surgical simulators and simulated surgeons: Reconstituting medical practice and practitioners in simulations. *Social Studies of Science, 37*(4), 585–608. https://doi.org/10.1177/0306312706072179.

Kemper, P. F., de Bruijne, M., van Dyck, C., So, R. L., Tangkau, P., Wagner, C. (2016). Crew resource management training in the intensive care unit. A multisite controlled before–after study. *BMJ Quality & Safety, 25*(8), 577–587. https://doi.org/10.1136/bmjqs-2015-003994.

Kolb, D. A. (1984). *Experiential learning: Experience as the source of learning and development*. Engelwood Cliffs: Prentice Hall.

Meurling, L., Hedman, L., Sandahl, C., Felländer-Tsai, L., Wallin, C. J. (2013). Systematic simulation-based team training in a Swedish intensive care unit: A diverse response among critical care professions. *BMJ Quality & Safety, 22*(6), 485–494. https://doi.org/10.1136/bmjqs-2012-000994. [Published Online First: 2013/02/16].

Meurling, L., Hedman, L., Lidefelt, K. J., Escher, C., Wallin, C. J. (2014). Comparison of high- and low equipment fidelity during paediatric simulation team training: A case control study. *BMC Medical Education, 14*(221). https://doi.org/10.1186/1472-6920-14-221. [Published Online First: 2014/10/20].

Mitchell, L., Flin, R., Yule, S., Mitchell, J., Coutts K., Youngson, G. (2013). Development of a behavioral marker system for scrub practitioners' non-technical skills (SPLINTS system). *Journal of Evaluation in Clinical Practice, 19*(2), 317–323. https://doi.org/10.1111/j.1365-2753.2012.01825.x.

Moffatt-Bruce, S. D., Hefner, J. L., Mekhjian, H. (2017). What is the return on investment for implementation of a crew resource management program at an academic medical center? *American Journal of Medical Quality, 32*(1), 5–11. https://doi.org/10.1177/1062860615608938.

Morey, J. C., Simon, R., Jay, G. D., Wears, L. R., Salisbury, M., Dukes, K. A., et al. (2002). Error reduction and performance improvement in the emergency department through formal teamwork training: Evaluation results of the medteams project. *Health Services Research, 37*(6), 1553–15581. https://doi.org/10.1111/1475-6773.01104.

Neily, J., Mills, P. D., Yinong, Y. X. (2010). Association between implementation of a medical team training program and surgical mortality (report). *JAMA, 304*(15), 1693.

Nestel, D., Kelly, M., Jolly, B., Watson, M. (2018). *Healthcare simulation education: Evidence, theory and practice.* New York: Wiley.

Nestel, D., Mobley, B. L., Hunt, E. A., Eppich, W. J. (2014). Confederates in health care simulations: Not as simple as it seems. *Clinical Simulation in Nursing, 10*(12), 611–616. https://doi.org/10.1016/j.ecns.2014.09.007.

Norman, G., Dore, K., Grierson, L. (2012). The minimal relationship between simulation fidelity and transfer of learning. *Medical Education, 46*(7), 636–647. https://doi.org/10.1111/j.1365-2923.2012.04243.x.

Nyström, S., Dahlberg, J., Hult, H. (2016). Enacting simulation: A sociomaterial perspective on students interprofessional collaboration. *Journal of Interprofessional Care, 30*(4), 441–447. https://doi.org/10.3109/13561820.2016.1152234.

O'Dea, A., O'Connor, P., Keogh, I. (2014). A meta-analysis of the effectiveness of crew resource management training in acute care domains. *Postgraduate Medical Journal, 90*(1070), 699. https://doi.org/10.1136/postgradmedj-2014-132800.

Østergaard, D., Dieckmann, P., Lippert, A. (2011). Simulation and CRM. *Best Practice & Research Clinical Anaesthesiology, 25*(2), 239–249. https://doi.org/10.1016/j.bpa.2011.02.003.

Oxelmark, L., Nordahl Amorøe, T., Carlzon, L., Rystedt, H. (2017). Students' understanding of teamwork and professional roles after interprofessional simulation-a qualitative analysis. *Advances in Simulation, 2*(8). https://doi.org/10.1186/s41077-017-0041-6.

Paige, J. B., & Morin, K. H. (2013). Simulation fidelity and cueing: A systematic review of the literature. *Clinical Simulation in Nursing,* (11), e481–e89. https://doi.org/10.1016/j.ecns.2013.01.001.

Parsh, B. (2010). Characteristics of effective simulated clinical experience instructors: Interviews with undergraduate nursing students. *Journal of Nursing Education, 49*(10), 569–572.

Patterson, M. D., Geis G. L., LeMaster, T., Wears R. L. (2013). Impact of multidisciplinary simulation-based training on patient safety in a paediatric emergency department. *BMJ Quality & Safety, 22*(5), 383–393. https://doi.org/10.1136/bmjqs-2012-000951.

Pierre, M. S. (2011). *Crisis management in acute care settings.* Berlin: Springer.

Robinson, A., & Mania, K. (2007). Technological research challenges of flight simulation and flight instructor assessments of perceived fidelity. *Simulation & Gaming, 38*(1), 112–135. https://doi.org/10.1177/1046878106299035.

Ruesseler, M., Weinlich, M., Müller, M. P., Byhan, C., Marzi, I., Walcher, F. (2012). Republished: Simulation training improves ability to manage medical emergencies. *Postgraduate Medical Journal, 88*(1040), 312–316. https://doi.org/10.1136/pgmj-2009-074518rep.

Rystedt, H., & Sjöblom, B. (2012). Realism, authenticity, and learning in healthcare simulations: Rules of relevance and irrelevance as interactive achievements. *Instructional Science, 40*(5), 785–798. https://doi.org/10.1007/s11251-012-9213-x.

Salas E., & Burke, C. S. (2002). Simulation for training is effective when .... *Quality and Safety in Health Care, 11*(2), 119–120. https://doi.org/10.1136/qhc.11.2.119.

Wallin, C.-J., Meurling, L., Felländer-Tsai, L. (2009). ATEAM: Targets for training, feedback and assessment of all OR members teamwork. In R. Flin, & L. Mirchell (Eds.), *Safer surgery* (1st edn). Ashgate publishing group.

WHO. (2009). *WHO patient safety curriculum guide for medical schools.*

Yule, S., Flin, R., Maran, N., Rowley, D., Youngson, G., Paterson-Brown, S. (2008). Surgeons' non-technical skills in the operating room: Reliability testing of the NOTSS behavior rating system. *World Journal of Surgery, 32*(4), 548–556. https://doi.org/10.1007/s00268-007-9320-z.Rue.

4.4 Commentary

Håkan Hult
Karolinska Institutet
Stockholm, Sweden
email: hakan.hult@ki.se

The chapter focuses on the facilitator's situation during briefing and simulation. Husebø and Rystedt study how the facilitator acts when briefing students, and this is something that is rarely investigated. I agree with their conclusion that:

The results of the study emphasize the tacit, often taken for granted aspects of instructions and points to the briefing as a much more complex and critical to the simulation scenario than presented in simulation textbooks and research.

One of Husebø and Rystedt's major contributions is the analytical approach they use, interaction analysis (IA). The method is used to study how people interact with each other and with artifacts in their surroundings. By studying the interaction in the smallest detail, Husebø and Rystedt help us to draw attention to situations the facilitator faces when briefing students and how the facilitator chooses to act. The facilitator can choose to focus the briefing only on informing about the scenario and showing the students the simulation facilities or the facilitator can also choose to teach the students when needed. Staff need to practice technical and non-technical skills while students need both to practice and learn. This can make the facilitator's roll more complex when briefing students. In Husebø and Rystedt's study the facilitator chooses to teach both about things he/she perceives the students do not know enough about and the gap between simulation realism and healthcare reality.

Husebø and Rystedt study just nursing students and thus there is no interprofessional simulation being studied. The facilitator's possibilities and conditions for teaching during briefing differs depending on the participants. Had the facilitator taught in a different way, about different things or not taught at all during the briefing, if there had been both nurse students and medical students participating in the simulation?

Escher et al. also focus on something that is rarely studied namely forms for the extra scenario information that the facilitator can provide during simulation-based team work training (SBTT). Simulation simulate healthcare and clinical practice, but the environment and the artifacts are not exactly what the participants are used to, for example the manikins have deficiencies; they cannot talk, the skin is not like real skin, etc. Therefore, the facilitator sometimes needs to give extra information, and that can be done in many ways. Escher et al. discuss the pros and cons of each method for in-scenario instruction. A weakness they raise is that an information delay results in declining pace. When the participants work with the scenario they are in a "bubble" (the simulation reality), and it is important that they can remain in the "bubble" throughout the simulation. This is why the methods for and timing of the facilitator's additional information is important, sensitive and in need of much more research.

Is high-tech always better than low-tech? It is reasonable to think that the effect of the simulation will be better if the room and the artifacts are as realistic as possible, but there is a discussion going on about the value of high fidelity for motivation and learning. Escher et al. contribute to this discussion with a study where they found that the value for the participants of the SBTT can be the same regardless of the level of manikin fidelity. The level of fidelity seems to be most important to the facilitator since he/she must be more observant and alert when using a low fidelity manikin.

Chapter 5
Doing Interprofessional Simulation

Nick Hopwood, Song-ee Ahn, Sanna Rimpiläinen, Johanna Dahlberg, Sofia Nyström, and Ericka Johnson

5.1 Introduction

Nick Hopwood
University of Technology Sydney
Sydney, Australia

University of Stellenbosch
Stellenbosch, South Africa
email: nick.hopwood@uts.edu.au

What does it mean to do interprofessional simulation? Such a seemingly simple and innocent question is unpacked in this chapter to reveal its beguiling nature. In this introduction my aim is to provide readers with cues, suggestions and tantalising glimpses, in the hope that these might foster a reading that is aligned with the authors' intended terms of engagement, and which draws out meanings and connections that might otherwise have been less obvious. Both sections offer analyses informed by sociomaterial theory, exploring how the doing of interprofessional

N. Hopwood (✉)
University of Technology Sydney, Sydney, Australia

University of Stellenbosch, Stellenbosch, South Africa
e-mail: nick.hopwood@uts.edu.au

S.-e. Ahn · J. Dahlberg (✉) · S. Nyström · E. Johnson
Linköping University, Linköping, Sweden
e-mail: song.ee.ahn@liu.se; johanna.dahlberg@liu.se; sofia.nystrom@liu.se;
ericka.johnson@liu.se

S. Rimpiläinen
University of Strathclyde, Glasgow, Scotland
e-mail: sanna.rimpilainen@dhi-scotland.com

© Springer Nature Switzerland AG 2019
M. Abrandt Dahlgren et al. (eds.), *Interprofessional Simulation in Health Care*,
Professional and Practice-based Learning 26,
https://doi.org/10.1007/978-3-030-19542-7_5

simulation emerges in fluid relationships between different (human and nonhuman) actors. What follows highlights features of each, and connections between them in terms of multiplicity, messiness, and medicine.

Sociomaterial analyses resist reductive accounts of a singular 'truth', opening up instead to multiplicity. Anh and Rimpiläinen's work reminded me of Massey's (2005) ideas of space as a coming together of (multiple) trajectories or stories-so-far. In their account, the gaze is widened to incorporate spaces away from action around the simulator, and the entangling and coalescing of unfolding trajectories between them is clearly laid out. This is infused with another layer of multiplicity – that of knowings. Dahlberg and Nyström elucidate a multiplicity of simulated bodies, in which Mol's (2002) work on "real" patients' bodies comes to mind. They reveal a(nother!) multitude of more or less choreographed bodily assemblages, anticipations, and responses among the learners.

Just as sociomaterial accounts resist reductionism, they also resist the imposition or even expectation of coherence and linearity. Embracing mess reframes the analysis in helpful ways. Learning through simulation emerges in this chapter as both ruled and unruly. Ruled by social norms, pedagogic norms, curricular intentions, and technological affordances. But these rulings do not determine the unfolding practices. We see unruly intrusions – look out for injurious intubation, affect and sweating bodies, missed care for a head, the inscrutable manikin, and untended wounds.

Medicine provides a third productive point of connection between the sections that follow. Medical knowings are not limited to knowledge of the body and treatment, but also revealed in their performative aspects around (becoming) professionals' bodily positionings, and movements, and the things of medicine (look for the torch). Medical bodies appear in simulated form, requiring more than the simulator to take on this meaning, colliding with human bodies (look out for a tucked blanket). Medicine also forms trajectories of practice that synchronise (or not) with those of nursing. We can take this chapter as a basis to understand medicine and the medical in challenging but exciting ways.

Contributions to this book share a commitment to understanding simulation not as an end in itself, but as a means to foster learning. The literature of simulation as educational tool is striking in its largely normative and prescriptive nature. Both sections in this chapter show how learning emerges through but also in spite of the enactment of plans that follow dominant prescriptions of 'good' simulation pedagogy. Interprofessional learning is indeed shaped by curriculum, scenarios, technologies, facilitator prompts and questions. But ruptures also emerge, and I encourage readers to seek out ghostly anticipations, unmet urgencies, deviations, spontaneous eruptions or closures of possibility (look for the technical breakdown). Through these, we can see how, for all possible prefiguration, fluid assemblages of the human and nonhuman defy complete control: learning remains deliciously open, unfinished and unruly.

References

Massey, D. (2005). *For space*. London: Sage.
Mol, A. (2002). *The body multiple: Ontology in medical practice*. London: Duke University Press.

5.2   Location and Knowings

Song-ee Ahn
Linköping University
Linköping, Sweden
email: song.ee.ahn@liu.se

Sanna Rimpiläinen
University of Strathclyde
Glasgow, Scotland
email: sanna.rimpilainen@dhi-scotland.com

5.2.1   Introduction

This chapter treats simulation as a means to fostering learning. We examine how learning and knowing emerge in the different locations – the simulation, control and reflection rooms – involved in the simulation training. The focus is on the varying socio-material assemblages in these locations and how they coalesce or fall apart affecting learning and knowing by the participants.

A number of meta-analyses of simulation studies (e.g. Cant and Cooper 2010; Cook et al. 2011) have shown that high technology-enhanced simulation training has a significant positive effect on learning, knowledge, skills and behaviour of medical and nursing students. Simulation training is also seen to be important teaching method to increase group performance, interprofessional communication and understanding, as well as satisfaction and confidence among the participants. High fidelity simulators are regarded to be especially suited for training students (and professionals) not only in technical and medical skills but also in non-technical skills such as team-building, leadership, communication and decision-making (e.g. Eich et al. 2007). Considering that communication between different groups of professionals in health care have been identified as significant in medical practices (Barr et al. 2005), high technology-enhanced simulation seems to be answer for various challenges in medical education. While there is a large body of knowledge that supports the view that high technology-enhanced simulation in health education is an effective teaching method, there is still lack of knowledge focusing on the process of students' learning and how knowledge emerges and manifests itself in the simulation training, which this chapter concerns.

5.2.2   Knowing as Enactment

In this chapter we investigate "doings" and the types of knowing that emerge in the different locations involved in simulation training (see also Ahn et al. 2015). For analysis we have drawn upon an approach that belongs to the family of practice-oriented theories (see Chap. 2) useful for studying human-technology relations, Actor-Network Theory (ANT).The approach provides tools for analysing socio-materiality and disentangling how practices and their effects emerge – on this occasion, in a pedagogical setting (e.g. Fenwick and Edwards 2010; Law 2004; Latour 2005). Principles that guide ANT analyses can seem radical from the traditional social sciences' point of view.

Firstly, ANT argues that both humans and nonhumans can "act". ANT treats materiality, non-human actors, as equal participants in practices: the simulator is an as important actor in the exercise as are the students or their teachers. However, ANT makes a distinction between intentional action, and acting by "affecting states of affairs": objects "act" through being entangled in networks or assemblages with other actors (Callon 1986; Latour 2005). This is the way in which the simulator acts: it necessarily influences states of affairs as part of the socio-material entanglement that comes together to produce the simulation exercise. This chapter provides several examples of this.

Secondly, ANT departs from the traditional worldview which stipulates that the world, our reality, is something that simply exists out-there, ready to be observed. Instead, the world is seen as emergent, and as enacted into being through the different doings engaged by conglomerations of human and non-human actors. In other words, materiality and the social are inseparable from one another in producing the realities we live in. (e.g. Callon 1986; Fenwick and Edwards 2010; Law 2004; Latour 2005).

The main focus of this chapter is the concept of "knowing" (how you come to "know" something). ANT does not regard the phenomenon either as a cognitive or a social one (e.g. Sørensen 2009). Knowing emerges as an effect of the socio-material arrangements that gather together and are performed into being through the continual transactions, which are part of the practice (Law 2009; Rimpiläinen 2011; Sørensen 2009). In other words, knowing is an enactment. The crux of the concept of enactment is that these take place in physical locations, such as the simulation room at a hospital, and that they are inextricable from "doing". Enactments are achieved in, by and through the relationships among the diverse entities in those physical locations (Law 2009) Therefore, knowing as an enactment can be taken as a local and a temporal product. To understand how "knowing" emerges as part of the simulation, it is crucial to know which practices and which socio-material entanglements are involved in the process.

In this chapter, we follow the simulator as a focal actor in order to elaborate and understand how the patient Anna becomes enacted into being (or not) during the simulation exercises. Focusing analytically on the simulator enables us to zoom in on the "doings" taking place, who and what are involved in these doings, and crucially, what the *effects* of these assemblages and doings are (Mol 2002; Rimpiläinen 2012). By approaching phenomena following the principles of ANT, we shift the singular focus on human – customary in social science research – to *associations of human and nonhuman actors*, and upon the effects such assemblages have e.g. on producing and affecting our day-to-day practices. ANT also helps us resist landing upon a singular truth, but helps us trace multiple, sometimes competing, realities.

5.2.3 *Locations and Materials of the Simulation*

5.2.3.1 Locations

The simulation training discussed in this chapter involves three different locations; simulation, control and reflection rooms (Ahn et al. 2015). The first location is the *simulation room* itself. The simulation training was arranged for mixed groups of nursing and medical students in the last semester of their education, with the purpose of carrying out full-scale simulations of acute trauma handling. The simulation room was furnished as an emergency room with medicines, medical equipment, furniture, an oxygen tank, gloves, a telephone, drips and computer monitors. In addition, there was a one-way window to the *control room*, which is the second location. The manikin functions through being connected to a computer run by an operator in the control room. The briefing preceding the exercise was done in both locations as the teachers and the operator informed the students about the scenario and materials/equipment involved in the exercise. All students could not participate in the simulation, partly because of lack of time and resources, partly due to large group sizes. Therefore, the students were divided into two groups: a team of five would participate in the exercise in the simulation room, with the rest of the students observing it in the control room with the medical teacher and the operator. The control room had a desk with a computer and three monitors; one displayed a silhouette of the manikin showing its bodily functions, while the other monitors showed the simulation room from different angles. There was a row of stools for the observers to occupy at the back of the room, giving a good view of the simulation room through the one-way window and through the monitor displays. Those in the control room could hear what was going on in the simulation room, but not vice-versa. The third location was a *meeting room* for debriefing following the simulation, where the student team that performed simulation and the students who observed the simulation gathered together to reflect upon the simulation. This room was furnished with small tables and comfortable chairs.

5.2.3.2 Scenario and the Simulator

This section describes two specifics "things" or actors that brought the simulation exercise to life: the scenario and the simulator (Ahn et al. 2015). The scenario involved a young car accident victim, a 17-year old girl, Anna. The scenario had two elements: the medical case that was presented to the students, and another one that was embedded in the exercise.

The simulation exercise began with a briefing, during which the students were informed that Anna had been found unconscious at the scene of the accident, but that she had grunted a little during the transport to the hospital. She had no visible injuries except for some bleeding on the left side of her head. The ambulance staff had given her some oxygen and a neck-collar to protect her neck. This was all the information the students were given.

The embedded learning element would emerge during the exercise, provided the students followed the mandated medical procedure for treating an acute trauma case – the so called the "ABCDE" routine: to check Airways (Stage A), Breathing (Stage B), Circulation (Stage C), Do a neurological check-up (Stage D) and Exposure and environmental control (Stage E). If the teams followed the routine and repeatedly performed the different stages of the procedure each time a change in the patient's condition was detected, they would discover that Anna's condition was deteriorating rapidly, and that they needed to call for help engaging different colleagues from around the hospital.

The manikin has different configurations. The medical actions enabled by this version of the manikin included measuring the pulse, taking temperature, giving oxygen, inserting a catheter or inserting a drip on a patient's vein. The manikin is immobile, but it can be lifted and moved around. As the simulator it cannot respond to touch, the students received this type of information, such as the patient's reactions to stimuli, via a loudspeaker from the control room, where the simulator was being operated from. Additionally, the manikin's pupils could be changed manually, so that these altered in size. This was a crucial element of the simulation, as that indicated a change in the patient's condition.

5.2.4   Knowings and Locations

The empirical material for this chapter was generated through observing 15 rounds of full-scale simulations of acute trauma in undergraduate education of health professionals in Sweden. The exercises were carried out by mixed groups of nursing and medical students. Each group was divided into two subgroups; a group of four-five students performed the simulation and the others observed the simulation from the control room. A research team of four members attended three training days. Each observation was carried out by two researchers, one taking notes in the simulation room, the other in the observation/control room. Both researchers attended the debriefing session following each simulation. Five of the simulation sessions were also video-recorded. Repeated observations of the repeated runs of the structured simulation exercise taking place in the same setting have allowed for a pattern or a "usual" sequence of events to emerge. This has enabled us to compare the different types of effects that have arisen as a result of the changing assemblages of the human and nonhuman in the different locations. (For more information about the study see Ahn et al. 2015).

The following section presents our main findings (Ahn et al. 2015). Through repeated rounds of observation of the simulation exercises, we discovered the emergence of different types of knowings: *medical knowing, affective knowing and communication*. These knowings made appearance in all three locations. However, due to the divergent socio-material entanglements in all three, the knowings emerged in different forms. The exercise that took place in the simulation room had dual function: we analysed it as a setting where different knowings emerged, while the exercise also became material for observation, analysis and reflection in the other two locations involved in the simulation. This is also the reason why the description of the simulation room is given more space in this article than the other two locations.

5.2.4.1 Simulation Room

As a pedagogical space, the simulation room is a location for learning by doing. It is important to understand that there was an intended learning path embedded in the scenario used in the simulation and that it could only be followed when the team enacted the scenario as if the situation was for real, and therefore demonstrated their medical knowings as part of it.

The teams were encouraged to do "...whatever they needed to do as interns", and act as if they were in a real emergency situation, with the simulator a patient whose life they needed to save. The teams that were successful in enacting the simulator as the patient Anna and in following the intended learning path started immediately to act as if they really were working as interns at an emergency ward, preparing for the arrival of an acute trauma patient. From the word go, they would, for example, put on plastic aprons and gloves, and prepare medical equipment for the arrival of the patient. The most significant marker of the team's engagement with the scenario as-if-it-was-for-real was how they related to the simulator: for example, did the team talk to the simulator as they would to a real patient, or did they talk *about* the simulator like a piece of equipment? Teams that did the former usually approached the simulator saying things like "Anna, you are now at the hospital, you have been in a car accident. I am doctor and will take care of you." These types of actions show how medical knowing emerges in the simulation site: through the team's performance related to the materiality of the simulation room, and through "suspending disbelief" (Essington 2010) and the treatment of the "as if" of the exercise as "as is". When the team succeeded in suspending disbelief during the simulation, this would also manifest itself when the team had to handle a vomiting patient that was wearing a neck rest. Here the test was whether the team would take care of the patient's head when turning the head to one side. For the simulator it made no difference whether its head was being supported during the turn or not; for the patient this would be crucially important. Another test arose when the team would discover the altered pupil size in the patient's eye following the first completed round of the ABCDE-routine: the dilated pupil indicating a life-threatening change in the patient's condition, signalling raised intracranial pressure and uncal herniation. Actions that arose following this discovery also manifested the levels of medical knowing by the teams.

What is important to point out is that not all actions or doings taking place during the exercise were related to the intended learning path. Students *could* do many different things, such as intubate Anna, even though she was breathing normally, or insert a tube into Anna's nose. These actions did not hurt the simulator, but they would have been dangerous to be performed on a patient with a head injury. The way the teams related and interacted with the scenario and the materiality of the simulation room highlighted the level of their medical proficiency (Ahn and Rimpiläinen 2018).

The moment that the team picked up a unilaterally dilated pupil in the patient's eye kicked off the most stressful part of the simulation exercise: the team faced a real emergency. At that moment the mood in the room often changed and a particular form of *affective knowing,* entailing expressing and handling feelings, values and emotions, emerged. This had to do with the emotional aspect of working in a high-pressure situation trying to save a patient's life and making decisions quickly and decisively. Handling that level of stress was an important experience. During many of the exercises we observed, it was obvious that team were experiencing high levels of stress and anxiety, uncertainty, sometimes even shame as well as pride. The students reported these emotions manifesting themselves as physical, bodily experiences such as sweating, sweaty and shaky hands, stomach pains, drying mouth, inability to think clearly etc. The emotions and reactions to the simulated situation were something that the students had not expected to experience during the exercise. At the same time, handling stress reactions like these is not something that can be learned by reading textbooks. The physical reactions also showed the degree to which the teams managed to suspend disbelief, and enact the simulator as a real-life patient, whose life was at risk, while in reality there was no human patient who could die as a result of the actions of the team.

The third form of knowing that emerged in the simulation room was *communication.* The purpose of the simulation exercise was to support interprofessional learning. The exercise was in the last semester of both medical and nursing programs, and it was the very first time the students from these programs worked together. Even if doctors and nurses would work side by side in their future professional lives, their education is separated. The ability for smooth interprofessional working has been pointed out as an important aspect for patient safety. The affordances of the manikin, what it can and cannot do, are important for the simulation and its pedagogical purposes. The fact that the manikin is unable to display any bodily reactions necessitates the doctors examining Anna to state clearly what they are doing at any given moment in order to receive any medical information from the operator. These theatrical and unrealistic actions are comprehensible within the site of the exercise, and necessary for the simulation to carry on. It is also a way for the whole team to *communicate* and *share* information on the patient in a very specific way. The affordances of the manikin enforced clear communication not only between the team and the staff in the control room but also among the team members. The necessity for clear and effective communication is not at stake only between the team members (between doctors and nurses) but also between the team at the Emergency room and the other professions at the hospital (played by the operator and the medical teacher in the control room). During the scenario the teams were expected to call for assistance. Trying to get hold of an anaesthetist was one of the most important parts of the scenario in terms of effective communication. The exercise made it clear that if the doctor was not able to communicate the urgency and the nature of the situation clearly enough to the other person on the phone, whose own medical priorities were taking precedence in their mind, the arrival of the anaesthetist would be delayed with dire consequences.

In the simulation room, the different types of knowings – medical knowing, affective knowing and communication- were dependent on students' ability to suspend disbelief and act as if the situation was real. Within the material set up of simulation room, there were actions that were medically (in)appropriate and (im)possible. The ability to suspend disbelief and act as if the situation was real means therefore that the team would act *medically appropriately* for the type of injury and patient in question, even though sometimes their action would be artificial and only understandable for those involved in simulation training. For example, stating "I'll put on some lubricant" before rectal examination would not be necessary in an emergency room, but is necessary for the simulation to continue. The enactment of the patient was a result of the team's engagement in enactment of the scenario as if it was a real case. It necessitated that students not only used the available materials but engaged each other and worked with them in specific ways that were understandable and acceptable as part of the simulation (Ahn and Rimpiläinen 2018).

5.2.4.2   Control Room

Control room was a space where students unable to participate in the simulation exercise observed the unfolding events accompanied by the medical teacher and the operator. They would sit in a school-like setting, observing the team's performance like a piece of theatre via a one-way window and three monitors that focused on the different aspects of the exercise. They could also see and hear how the teacher and the operator participated in enacting the scenario.

The most significant material for learning in this site was the performance that the students observed. Observation, not simply "seeing", is an action rooted in the practice that it takes place in. To understand what to observe, and how to understand what is being observed, the students need to understand simulation, and of its concerns, as a medical educational practice (cf. Latour 1987). From the first moments of the exercise, the medical teacher guided and structured the students' observations by instructing them to follow the team's medical actions and their communication, or the medical comments they made during the simulation. The medical teacher played different roles: whenever she entered the simulation room, she was a colleague (from somewhere else in the hospital) to the Emergency team, but while she was in the Control room, she was a teacher to the students. She tried to actively involve the students in the Control room with questions such as "At which stage are they now?", and with comments, such as" They did not take care of her head". The students could ask questions at any time during the simulation, and the teacher would often give them extra information about the situation, explaining how the patient was expected to react, or why they did not do as expected. They would also explain what different symptoms indicated in medical terms, while at the same time only giving descriptive information of symptoms to the team in the simulation room.

Affective learning for the students in the Control was also different. While they could not experience the affective side of being medical professionals trying to save a patient's life in an acute situation first-hand, they experienced what they observed. Some of the students could relate to the team's emotional experiences as observers. Later, the team's simulation become material for group discussions, questions and reflections.

If simulation could be described as performance, the control room was a backstage. The hidden part of scenario was present throughout the simulation. Beside the running commentaries on the team's performance, the observers could also see how the medical teacher and operator gave answers and communicated as a part of the wider "hospital", which the emergency room had access to via a telephone. When the team discovered the dilated pupil, they would call for support. Usually the doctor in the simulation room is looking for an anaesthetist, but it was always a midwife they had to talk to instead. The midwife (played by the Operator) would not want the anaesthetist (the Teacher) to leave for the emergency room before she had finished treating his patient. As long as the doctor did not require to talk with the anaesthetist directly, the midwife would offer to deliver a message. The operator, as the midwife, would summarize the message to be delivered but with missing important facts. While only the doctor in the simulation room could participate in this conversation, all students in the control room shared the whole conversation. More significantly, the operator and the medical teacher would explain why the conversation went in that specific way; people would not let the specialist go if it was not obvious that it concerned an emergency. Further, they explained how to deliver a message and the importance of checking that the other part understood the message. The case gave the students important lessons on how to communicate interprofessionally within the different practices in the hospital.

As a pedagogical site the control/observation room can be described as a unique combination of classroom, panopticon, backstage and the extension of the manikin as mind and bodily reactions of Anna (Ahn et al. 2015). The medical and affective knowing in this location emerged as discursive rather than experiential learning. While the simulation team performed their knowing by doing, both the medical and affective knowings in the Control room were performed discursively, sitting side-by-side in a classroom-like situation, supported and guided by a teacher. By asking the relevant medical questions and providing the relevant answers to the teacher when she asked, by discussing happenings in the simulation as material for learning, the students' knowing emerged. Communication here had more tutorial character; the medical feedback on what the team in the simulation room were given in this room by the teacher. It was also spontaneous, including teacher's answers and comments, and sometimes quite critical noting which mistakes the team may have made.

5.2.4.3   The Reflection Room

The simulation exercise always had a happy ending: Anna's life was saved, and she moved on to other parts of the hospital. The simulator returned to be a simulator. All students, the teachers and the operator moved to a conference room for debriefing. In this site, seated in a circle with their professional clothes on, they reflected upon the simulation. Those who had engaged in the simulation talked about their experiences of it, how they had taken decisions and what they felt while taking care of the patient. The observer-students could comment on the simulator team's actions and professional behaviours and discuss how the team communicated and made decisions. In this space, the students were colleagues and the teachers were moderators of the discussion. Medical knowing was enacted in a discursive and reflective way. The team's performance became material for discussion, something that they could detach themselves from and that they could learn from. The Anna/manikin, as a physical object, was not present in the reflection site but the *effect* of her/it was there as a material for learning.

The affective aspect of simulation was one of the main discussion themes. While the simulation team described and shared their emotional experiences – something that had often come as a surprise to them – the observers contributed to discussion with their interpretations and observations on how the team had handled the situation, and how they might do better the next time. The teaching staff often shared their experiences and gave advice, such as the importance of the ABCDE structure, or using a notebook during an acute case.

Communication in the reflection room was characterized by a collegium. It might not be surprising that the observer-students changed their communication style most strikingly, when they were together with the team face to face. During the simulation, the students were separated, and therefore there was an appropriate distance between the team performing and the team observing. The comments made about the performance were perhaps more critical and more spontaneous. In the reflection room, both teams were together as colleagues, whose actions and decisions required understanding and respect. The focus was on collegial professional communication: how best to discuss and constructively comment on decisions and actions taken by one's peers? The teaching staffs also took this collegial role in the reflection room: rather than pointing out any medical mistakes made in the simulation, they waited for someone to mentioned them. Otherwise mistakes were not taken up for discussion in the reflection room.

5.2.5 Conclusion

In this section, we have explored a setting for interprofessional learning, where the human participants have inhabited different roles and held different responsibilities. Our approach, however, has allowed us to transcend these roles and responsibilities and focus upon not only what the students learned but also on how the learning took place: how the different "doings" as part of the varying socio-material constellations of each location enabled different ways of learning as well as the emergence of different types of knowing (Fenwick and Edwards 2010; Rimpilainen 2011; Sørensen 2009). The shifting socio-material arrangements in the three sites conditioned, guided, afforded and anticipated divergent actions and doings for learning. All three locations were pedagogical sites and the three types of knowing were observed in all three, but they were enacted in different ways.

The chapter highlights the importance of materiality in planning the pedagogical journey for the students. What traditional social science might deem as a "social" outcome, something that emerges solely from human interaction, is in fact a result of careful manipulation of the available materiality in the learning locations within which the humans find themselves. The materiality in the three locations guided, even dictated, the way in which students and the teaching staffs engaged with each other, with the learning matter, the simulator, how they were able to participate and contribute to the exercise, and how they learned. While the different material arrangements in the simulation were created with a particular pedagogical intention in mind, these could also in turn create boundaries for propriety – for what kinds of actions were possible, acceptable and understandable for those involved in each location (see Ahn and Rimpiläinen 2018).

- All three simulation locations – the simulation, the control and the reflection room – are important pedagogical spaces but the nature of knowing and learning outcomes differ.
- The article highlights the importance of considering the materiality in planning pedagogical journeys for students, and how manipulating the scenario and socio-material settings of the simulation can impact learning outcomes.
- The socio-material arrangements made available in the different locations enable as well as de-limit possible (acceptable for the situation) types of actions, roles and communications.
- Approaching an interprofessional training session through Actor Network Theory has enabled us to transcend the differences between medical and nursing students, and instead focus on jointly performed practices, and the emergent effects of that activity. This has offered a fresh way to examine how learning takes place during a simulation exercise.

References

Ahn, S-E., Rimpiläinen, S., Theodorsson, A., Fenwick, T., Abrandt Dahlgren, M. (2015). Learning in technology enhanced medical simulation: Locations and knowings. *Professions and Professionalism, 5*(1), 1–12.
Ahn, S-E., Rimpiläinen, S. (2018). Maintaining Sofia – or how to reach the intended learning outcomes during a medical simulation training. *International Journal of Learning Technology, 13*(2), 115–129.
Barr, H., Koppel, I., Reeves S., Hammick, M., Freeth, D. (2005). *Effective interprofessional education*. Malden: Blackwell Publishing.
Callon, M. (1986). Some elements of a sociology of translation: domestication of the scallops and the fishermen of St Brieuc Bay. In J. Law (Ed.), *Power, action, and belief: A new sociology of knowledge* (pp.196–223). London: Routledge & Kegan Paul.
Cant, R.P., Cooper, S.J. (2010). Simulation-based learning in nurse education: systematic review. *Journal of Advanced Nursing, 66*(1), 3–15.

Cook, D.A., Hatala, R., Brydges, R., Zendejas, B., Szostek, J.H., Wang, A.T., et al. (2011). Technology-enhanced simulation for health professions education: a systematic review and meta-analysis. *The Journal of American Medical Association, 306*(9), 978–988.

Eich, A., Timmermann, A., Russo, S.G., Nickel, E.A. (2007). Simulator-based training in paediatric anaesthesia and emergency medicine –Thrills, skills and attitudes. *British Journal of Anaesthesia, 98*(4), 417–419.

Fenwick, T., & Edwards, R. (2010). *Actor-network theory in education.* London: Routledge.

Latour, B. (1987). *Science in Action.* Cambridge, MA: Harvard University Press.

Latour, B. (2005). *Reassembling the social: An introduction to actor-network theory.* Oxford: Oxford University Press.

Law, J. (2004). *After method: Mess in social science research.* Milton Park: Routledge.

Law, J. (2009). Actor network theory and material semiotics. In B. S. Turner (Ed.), *The new Blackwell companion to social theory, 3rd edition* (pp. 141–158). Chichester: Wiley-Blackwell.

Mol, A. (2002). *The body multiple: Ontology in medical practice.* Durham: Duke University Press.

Rimpiläinen, S. (2011). Knowledge in networks – knowing in transactions. *International Journal for Actor-Network Theory and Technological Innovation (IJANTTI), 3*(2), 45–56. doi: https://doi.org/10.4018/jantti.2011040104.

Rimpiläinen, S. (2012). *Gathering, translating, enacting. A study of interdisciplinary research and development practices in Technology Enhanced Learning.* (unpublished doctoral dissertation). Stirling: University of Stirling.

Sørensen, E. (2009). *The materiality of learning. Technology, knowledge in educational practice.* Cambridge, UK: Cambridge University Press.

5.3   Bodily Enactments in Interprofessional Simulation

Johanna Dahlberg · Sofia Nyström
Linköping University
Linköping, Sweden
email: johanna.dahlberg@liu.se; sofia.nystrom@liu.se

This section will problematise how interprofessional collaboration can be understood through a focus on different enactments of participating students. We will provide empirical analyses of how the social and material arrangements for interprofessional simulation produces different conditions for learning (Nyström et al. 2016). We argue that a focus on the emerging practice is useful to disentangle the complexity of simulation and has a potential to provide new knowledge on how interprofessional collaboration is played out in practice.

Previous studies have predominantly focused on participants' opinions of inter-professional simulation as a means of learning interprofessional collaboration, or as part of course evaluative frameworks (e.g. Alinier et al. 2014; Cook et al. 2011, Gough et al. 2012). Following a socio-material perspective on practices, our starting point is that practices are emergent, and situated to a specific location in time and space. This means that we are looking beyond taken-for-granted understandings of interprofessional collaboration and ways of conceptualising simulation as following a certain protocol. Instead, we ask: What is happening as students come together to practice interprofessional teamwork in simulated emergency scenarios? How is the unfolding practice related to the ways the simulation setting is arranged? According to Schatzki (2002), material arrangements prefigure the emerging practice. This means that material arrangements, for example in the emergency room, influence what will be performed, and consequently make some actions easier to take, or fol low, than others. Important for our analysis is also issues of corporeality, i.e. the significance and role of the enactment and positioning of bodies; the patient's body and the students' bodies as their interactions and collaborations unfold. Corporeality is regarded as an important dimension of what it means to be, to practice and to learn as a professional, that have implications for professional education (Green and Hopwood 2015). Recent theorisations of practice (Kinsella 2015) have suggested that a focus on the role of the body in professional practices, in simulated or natural-istic settings, might enable educators and learners to draw attention to other dimen-sions of knowledge, that are not easily accessible through cognitive perspectives, "dimensions that might help us illuminate, understand and investigate other types of knowledge that are relevant to everyday practices" (Kinsella 2015, p. 294).

As previously mentioned in Sect. 3.2, a cycle of simulation pedagogically follows three phases: briefing, simulation and debriefing. These phases have different socioma-terial arrangements and activities that encompass different challenges to educators and learners. The locations of the different phases of a simulation exercise are not just 'con-texts' or 'containers' where learning takes place (Ahn et al. 2015; see Sect. 5.2). In this section, we take the analysis of what is emerging during the unfolding scenario further, studying how the simulation scenario unfolds in practice (Nyström et al. 2016). Here we include a focus not only on the locations *per se*, but how the social and material arrange-ments for interprofessional simulation produces different conditions for learning.

This section builds on empirical analyses of video recordings from sessions where undergraduate nursing and medical students do simulation exercises that aimed to provide opportunities to practice professional skills as well as team-work and collaboration (Nyström et al. 2016). Students are introduced to differ-ent scenarios of emergency situations, where the condition could be unalarming in the beginning, but the patient is deteriorating as the scenarios progress. A purposeful approach to collaborative data analysis, comprising a layered process in three phases of activities (see Sect. 3.3), was utilised employing a field study approach. Ethnographic field studies have a long tradition of focusing on cultures and materiality and are also seen as in being in alignment with a sociomaterial perspective on practices (Fenwick et al. 2011; Schatzki 2012).

5.3.1 Enactments of the Patients' Body

Our findings show that students and student teams relate to the manikin in different ways as the scenario unfolds (Nyström et al. 2014, 2016). This means that students enact the manikin as multiple bodies, changing – depending on the issues raised in the scenario. Multiple enactments of the manikins' body were also found in a parallel project study by Hopwood et al. (2016; see Chap. 2). In the following, we will show how the manikin is enacted as a technical, a medical, and a human body, all of which are relevant and related to the development of the scenario. The ways students engaged with the manikin, and the tasks they were enacting reflected some of their specific professional roles and responsibilities but were also enacted as incentives to initiate or co-ordinate collaborative efforts. It was noticeable how students related to the manikin as a technical body, a medical body and a human body as the scenario was unfolding.

Enacting the manikin as a *technical body* was emerging in the briefing phase of the simulation, when the technical features and affordances of the manikin was presented. The technical body also came into play through the way's students performed the various examinations during the scenario in accordance with the affordances of the manikin. Examples of the adjustment of the examination to the technical body are the insertion of a peripheral venous catheter that needed to be performed on the right arm of the manikin. The briefing session also included the technical limitations for what could be physically examined. The manikin was breathing and answering to direct questions, but the inspection of injuries was impossible. The students were instructed to ask questions about the clinical data that they needed. The answers from the manikin and the clinical data was provided through a loudspeaker voice from the control room.

Students were also enacting the manikin as a *medical body* as the scenario unfolded. This enactment was foremost initiated by the medical students and were visible in the ways the clinical procedures were emerging. The theoretical medical knowings, of anatomical structures and the assessment of bodily functions in regard of injuries was displayed. Decisions followed by actions to ensure the medical status and safety of the manikin as a medical body.

A third way of enacting the manikin, as a *human body* emerged in the way students addressed the manikin as a person. Students were calling the manikin by the name of the patient in the scenario and informing her about what the next action of the team what supposed to include. The attunement to the manikin as a human body also showed the ways students were caring for the manikin. This enactment was foremost initiated by nursing students, and were visible in the ways the manikin, now patient, was cared for to make as comfortable as possible. Examples of this include touching the patient's arm while talking to her or tucking a blanket around the feet to keep her warm.

The ways students interacted with each other and the social and material arrangements of the situation showed how ATLS protocol (ABCDE) acted as an algorithm for the emerging teamwork, prioritizing attunement to the medical body over the human body. The protocol thereby also coordinated how the profession-specific roles and responsibilities were interfoliated with the interprofessional collaboration around the emerging events of the scenario. Our findings show how the manikin was enacted both as a piece of equipment and 'as if' it was a real patient.

According to Schatzki (2002), material arrangements prefigure emerging practice. The material arrangements in the emergency room make some actions easier to take or follow than others. Our data show that an unplanned technical failure in the equipment running the manikin prefigured the actions taken, defining the "as if" simulation situation as a de facto "as is" situation. An example of this is (site 1 – simulation 4) when the manikin/patient stopped breathing. All students dropped everything and focused on resuscitation. Then, in the speakers, students heard the instructor say, "The patient is breathing, so continue as first planned". This example shows how a technical breakdown of the simulator made the students react as if it was the human body failing. The instructors' comments re-directed the students' attunement to the predetermined, agreed up on scenario.

5.3.2 Interprofessional Collaboration as Knowings and Enactments

In this section, we will discuss how interprofessional collaboration can be understood through a focus on different enactments of participating students. We want to emphasise and recognise that the role of the body in knowledge production in practice since it goes beyond a focus on the individual practitioner. In line with Kinsella (2015), we will argue that the performance of a practice is constituted by the relational nature of material arrangements and professional bodies. Above we showed that nursing and medical students demonstrate their respective professional knowings in their enactments of the manikin as a medical and/or human body. In this section, we will discuss how interprofessional knowings and enactments were emerging as fluid movements. Below, we illustrate how these movements flow between *bodily positionings in synchrony* and *bodily positioning out of synchrony* in relation to the sociomaterial entities as well as the arrangement of the simulation room.

5.3.2.1 Bodily Positionings in Synchrony

The patient (the manikin), who has a head trauma after a car accident, starts to vomit. The medical student in charge of the patient directly steps up and secures the head and says, "We need to turn Anna. Position yourselves!". The second medical student and one of the nursing students move to the same side of the patient, secure the arm with the catheter and prepare to turn the patient. The medical student at the head then says 'On the count of three! One, two, three'. Simultaneously they turn Anna and the second nurse puts a bowl in front of Anna's mouth. The second medical student moves to the head and secures the airways. Once the patient is stabilized, still on her side, the second medical student moves again to investigate the back and spine for injuries, after which the patient is turned back to the original position. (Site 1 – simulation 3)

The transcribed video sequence above shows a chain of actions of interprofessional collaboration composed of different doings in interaction between the students. We argue in the study that when bodily positionings were in synchrony with the socio-material arrangements in interprofessional collaboration, the movements of the student team members were connected in a fluid chain of actions. The activities of the chain comprised *noticing* a sign indicating a deterioration of the patients' condition (auditory or visual), which was followed by enactment of leadership through *taking action or* responding through *attuning to the action of others*. In the attunement to the action of others, there was also *anticipation of the next action* in the way the material arrangements were related to (Nyström et al. 2016). For instance, when the medical student intended to test the eye reflexes, the nurse was handing over the torch, before the medical student had verbalized the intentions. The pattern of the collaboration is illustrated graphically in Fig. 5.1.

For the interprofessional collaboration to take place the study shows two important aspects how the leadership is taken, and how others respond. In the field note above, the leadership was executed when the patient's condition suddenly deteriorated, for instance when the unconscious patient starts to vomit. On a signal from one student, all members of the team reorganised their activities to one central purpose, to support the breathing of the patient. Here professional bodies are relating to each other in a manner described as "in sync", which demonstrates how the different activities are interrelated. When bodily positionings were in synchrony with the sociomaterial arrangements in interprofessional collaboration, the movements of the student team members were connected in a fluid chain of actions.

Another such example of leadership is how the nursing student in the team initiated hand wash and putting on gloves and disposable aprons while waiting for the patient to arrive in the ambulance transport. Without saying anything, all members on the team responded to her actions, as the actions reminded them that this is a scenario where we play the "full game".

These examples show how sayings and doings, as well as bodily movements are connected to materiality. The nursing and the medical students both enact their respective professional knowings and tasks in relation to the patient but through the synchronization of the bodily positions, their sayings and doings of the critical situation also enacts interprofessional knowings. The enactment of bodily positions in sync showed that when the medical students performed their tasks, such as palpating the pulse and reporting the rate, the nursing students anticipated the coming action by the medical students and handed them the necessary material equipment

Fig. 5.1 Interprofessional collaboration between nursing (N) and medical students (M) as bodily positionings in synchrony with sociomaterial arrangements

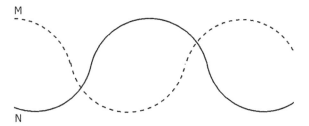

such as a torch or an oxygen mask. The interprofessional relationship between the medical and the nursing students was bundled with material entities, present or imagined in the location for the scenario.

The chain of action was composed of different doings in the interaction between the students. This continued until the patient was stabilized, and the members of the team turned back to the activities they had abandoned. Doing professional activities independently is described as "out of sync".

5.3.2.2 Bodily Positionings Out of Synchrony

When bodily positionings were out of synchrony with the sociomaterial arrangements, the fluidity of movements became disconnected by *task focused* performance and *dual agendas*. Noticing signs of deterioration and taking action did not lead to immediate attunement to the action of the others or responding through anticipation of the next step. Instead, the pattern of movements showed that parallel professional enactments without connection were taking place through the enactment of designated professional actions.

> *The nursing students stand in one corner of the room discussing how and when to prepare a urinary catheter. The two medical students stand in another corner of the room, looking for medical dosages in a drug compendium./.../After a while the medical students decide that the patient urgently needs to be transported to the X-ray room. The nursing students stop preparing the urinary catheter and help prepare the patient. (Site 1 – simulation 2)*

One example of this is in the field note above, where the nursing students and the medical students are separated in parallel professional enactments, both in their professional doings, sayings as well as physically in the room. Then the medical student takes the lead and the nurse student react to this despite that they cannot complete their planned action. By these sayings and doings, the chain of actions was eventually connected again by enactment of leadership, making dual agendas coalesce.

This type of interprofessional collaboration is also illustrated graphically in Fig. 5.2.

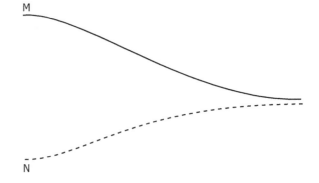

Fig. 5.2 Interprofessional collaboration between nursing (N) and medical students (M) as bodily positionings out of synchrony with sociomaterial arrangements. Dual agendas coalesce

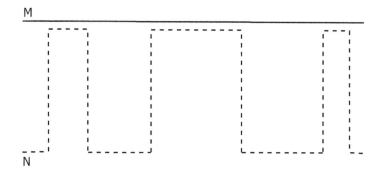

Fig. 5.3 Interprofessional collaboration between nursing (N) and medical students (M) as bodily positionings out of synchrony with sociomaterial arrangements. Both professional groups have a task focus

In our study, we saw other examples of bodily positionings being out of synchrony, how the participants were focusing on task-focused actions. In the field note below, a nursing and a medical student are going to suture a patient who has a wound on his leg. The medical student is all focused on following the protocol in a search for the problem. The nursing student is focused on the task given as well as preparing to take care of the patients' wound. This is another example where there are parallel professional enactments but in this example there are only brief moments of collaboration between the medical and the nursing students. This is illustrated graphically in Fig. 5.3

... come into the room and there is nothing 'alarming' about the patient, but the medical student directly starts to go through the procedure of ATLS, declaring that they have a clear airway, the lungs sound good and that they need to get a blood pressure reading. The nursing student tries to prompt the medical student that they need to suture the wound, but the medical student does not listen. The patient says, 'Why are you doing all these examinations on me? I'm not sick...'. The medical student answers 'No, no, we are just examining you and soon we are going to take care of your wound.'. She proceeds with her examinations following the ATLS protocol. The nursing student assists when requested, measuring the temperature etc. Otherwise the nursing student remains quiet but starts to prepare for the suture by arranging gloves and aprons, and a tray with syringe, anaesthetic and bandages. When the medical student has completed the examination according to the ATLS protocol she focuses on the wound and asks the patient if he has been anesthetized before. The patient does not really know. The medical student asks the nurse to bring out the adrenaline 'If something would happen...'. (Site 2 – simulation 3)

5.3.3   Discussion

In this section, we have applied a practice theory perspective on what is happening as students come together to enact interprofessional teamwork in simulated emergency scenarios. An important finding was how the students' knowing-in-practice was embodied and relational to the enactment of the manikin as body in different ways. The students shifted their attunement to the manikin/patient's body as being a technical, medical or human body. These shifts demonstrate how students' actions and interactions within the simulation are entangled with material arrangements. One plausible interpretation is also that the shifting attunements to different enactments of a medical or human body encompass possible fragments of professional perspectives of doctors and nurses in play. Students' attunement to the manikin/ patient as a technical body was intentionally related to the material arrangements of the simulation that required the participants to perform certain activities in ways that the technology allowed. However, the findings also demonstrate that the breakdown of the technical body the students to intentionally relate to the manikin as being a medical and human body.

Interprofessional collaboration in the simulation room was enacted as bodily positionings in and out of synchronization in a fluid way. Students' bodily positionings emerged in relation to the sociomaterial entities as well as the arrangements of the simulation room. When in sync, the students performed and enacted interprofessional collaboration where sayings, doings and bodily movements were connected in a chain of actions. Typically, when chains of actions were connected, and in sync, interprofessional collaboration emerged through the way they enacted their respective professional knowing in the context of others'. Participants were attuned to leading or responding to others' sayings and doings. When chains of actions were out of sync, the bodily movements were disconnected, creating parallel professional enactments. These findings could be related to what Johnson (2015), in a dynamic perspective on practice and practicing bodies, has described as 'enacted and embodied rhythms to practice' that generate a periodicity that enable practitioner to construct their practice together. There are multiple rhythms of various kinds in a practice, and these help the practitioners to sort the choices of actions undertaken. Johnson (2015) suggests that the sensitive synchronisation of practitioners' bodily actions and understandings is what shapes their professional practice.

5.3.4   Conclusions

The findings of this study can contribute to the development of simulation pedagogy for interprofessional learning with students. Bodily positionings direct educators' attention to the fluidity in movement. The articulation of bodily positionings in and out of synchrony can be used to disentangle the complexity of the interprofessional simulation and emphasize the collaborative part of the simulation. Bodily positionings were in synchrony when interprofessional collaboration was connected through noticing a sign indicating a deterioration of the patients' condition (auditory or visual), enactment of leadership through taking action, or responding through attuning to the action of others as well as anticipation of the next action of a peer student. Bodily positionings were out of synchrony when the fluidity in students' movements became disconnected by *task focused* individual performance and *dual agendas*. These phenomenons are related to contemporary theorisations of practice comprising an integrated view of body and mind. Being aware of this, designers of simulation exercises for interprofessional student teams should be able to support learning in new ways.

In this section, we have discussed that

- The student teams doing simulation relate to the manikin as a technical, medical, and human body, and that
- Interprofessional knowings and enactments emerge as a fluid movement between bodily positioning in synchrony and bodily positioning out of synchrony in relation to the sociomaterial arrangements.

References

Ahn, S-E., Rimpiläinen, S., Theodorsson, A., Fenwick, T. Abrandt Dahlgren, M. (2015). Learning in technology enhanced medical simulation: Locations and knowings. *Professions and Professionalism, 5*(1), 1–12.

Alinier, G., Harwood, C., Harwood, P., Montague, S., Huish, E., Ruparelia, K., Antuofermo, M. (2014). Immersive clinical simulation in undergraduate health care interprofessional education: Knowledge and perceptions. *Clinical Simulation in Nursing, 10*(4), e205–e216.

Cook, D.A., Hatala, R., Brydges, R., Zendejas, B., Szistek, J.K., Wang, A.T., Erwin, P.J., Hamstra, S.J. (2011). Technology-enhanced simulation for health professions education: A systematic review and meta-analysis. *JAMA, 7, 306*(9), 978–988.

Gough, S., Hellaby, M., Jones, N. MacKinnon, R. (2012). A review of undergraduate interprofessional simulation-based education. *Collegian, 19*(3), 153–171.

Green, B., Hopwood, N. (Eds.) (2015). *The body in professional practice, learning and education: Body/practice*. Dordrecht: Springer.

Fenwick, T., Edwards, R., Sawchuk, P. (2011). *Emerging approaches to educational research: Tracing the sociomaterial*. London: Routledge.

Hopwood, N., Kelly, M., Boud, D., Rooney, D. (2016). Simulation in higher education: A sociomaterial view. *Education Philosophy and Theory*. doi:https://doi.org /10.1080/00131857.2014.971403.

Johnson, M.C. (2015). Terroir and timespace: body rhythms in winemaking. In B. Green, & N. Hopwood, (Eds.), *The body in professional practice, learning and education: Body/practice* (pp. 71–88). Dordrecht: Springer.

Kinsella, E. A. (2015) Embodied knowledge: towards a corporeal turn in professional practice, research and education. In B. Green, & N. Hopwood, (Eds.) *The body in professional practice, learning and education: Body/practice* (pp. 245–261). Dordrecht: Springer.

Nyström, S., Dahlberg, J., Hult, H., Abrandt Dahlgren, M. (2014, 25–27 June). Crossing locations of enacting and observing simulations: Ways of constructing interprofessional learning. Paper presented at the Second International ProPEL conference 'Professional matters: Materialities and virtualities of professional learning', Stirling, UK.

Nyström, S., Dahlberg, J., Hult, H., Abrandt Dahlgren, M., (2016). Enacting simulation: A sociomaterial perspective on students' interprofessional collaboration. *Journal of Interprofessional Care, 30*(4), 441–447.

Schatzki, T. (2002). *The site of the social: A philosophical account of the constitution of social life and change.* University Park: Pennsylvania State University Press.

5.4   Commentary

Ericka Johnson
Linköping University
Linköping, Sweden
email: ericka.johnson@liu.se

At first glance, this chapter, *Doing interprofessional simulation*, would appear to focus on the 'doing', on the practices of enacting simulation and the richness available to analysis and learning when one pulls apart a simulation and asks questions about how it is done, how the communication between participants (especially those from different professional categories) is conducted, and what moments of rupture can offer participants and trainers.

But on closer reflection, the insights from this chapter are also very attuned to the material of the sociomaterial in simulations and the emergence of patient bodies and interprofessional communication around them in different contexts. Here the authors are inspired by Mol's work on multiple ontologies (Mol 2002), which speaks to how diseases and bodies can be enacted in difference sociomaterial constellations. The authors of this chapter engage praxiographical approaches to show how simulator bodies and medical needs are multiple and emergent.

The chapter begins with a contribution from Anh and Rimpiläinen which draws our attention to the places in which knowing emerges from simulator training. They bring us into the simulator room, the control room and the reflection room where debriefing occurs. Through close analysis of the discussions that occur in each, they show us how the simulated patient is enacted into being through sociotechnical assemblages – through looking at who and what are involved. Their close readings give voice to the way medical knowledge, affect and interprofessional communication are all forms of knowledge that emerge in the simulation.

In the second section of the chapter, Dahlberg and Nyström describe how student teams relate to the simulated manikin as a technical, medical and human body in fluid movements in and out of synchrony with the sociomaterial constellations of the simulation. Their work shows how important it is to consider affordances that the constellations of technologies and human bodies provide when examining the unfolding simulation. Here, too, the enactment of the patient is studied, with specific interest in the bodily positionings of human and nonhuman participants.

Both sections of this chapter engage with simulated bodies as sociomaterial actors. A fertile parallel to their approach can be found in Goodwin's work, which shows that the real patient body is also a sociomaterial actor (Goodwin 2009), a human-technical entanglement which requires interprofessional communication to read and know. Human patients are also mediated through technology, just as their simulated counterparts are. The agency of both is relational. One of the lessons drawn from research on the emergence of sociomaterial ontologies and the practices between human and nonhuman actors is the importance of analytically considering agential relationality. While ANT suggests that both human and nonhuman actors can be attributed agency, Suchman's reflections on this encourage us to remember that it matters where and how we draw the lines between humans and nonhumans (Suchman 2007). Viewing agency as relational prompts analytical interest in how it is produced, how it emerges. The work presented in this chapter shows what richness this theoretical approach can provide to studying interprofessional communication as it emerges around simulated (and by extension in non-simulated) sociomaterial, human-technical entanglements that we call patient bodies.

References

Goodwin, D. (2009). *Acting in anaesthesia. Ethnographic encounters with patients, practitioners and medical technologies.* Cambridge, UK: Cambridge University Press.

Mol, A. (2002). *The body multiple: Ontology in medical practice.* Durham: Duke University Press.

Suchman, L. (2007). *Human-machine reconfigurations. Plans and situated actions* (2nd ed.). Cambridge, UK: Cambridge University Press.

Chapter 6
Observing Interprofessional Simulation

**David Boud, Sofia Nyström, Madeleine Abrandt Dahlgren,
Johanna Dahlberg, Donna Rooney, Michelle Kelly, and Dara O'Keeffe**

6.1 Introduction

David Boud
Deakin University
Geelong, Australia

University of Technology
Sydney, Australia

Middlesex University
London, UK
e-mail: david.boud@uts.edu.au

D. Boud
Deakin University, Geelong, Australia

University of Technology, Sydney, Australia

Middlesex University, London, UK
e-mail: david.boud@uts.edu.au

S. Nyström · M. Abrandt Dahlgren · J. Dahlberg
Linköping University, Linköping, Sweden
e-mail: sofia.nystrom@liu.se; madeleine.abrandt.dahlgren@liu.se; johanna.dahlberg@liu.se

D. Rooney (✉)
University of Technology, Sydney, Australia
e-mail: donna.rooney@uts.edu.au

M. Kelly
Curtin University, Perth, Australia
e-mail: michelle.kelly@curtin.edu.au

D. O'Keeffe
Royal College of Surgeons in Ireland, Dublin, Ireland
e-mail: daraokeeffe@rcsi.ie

© Springer Nature Switzerland AG 2019
M. Abrandt Dahlgren et al. (eds.), *Interprofessional Simulation in Health Care*,
Professional and Practice-based Learning 26,
https://doi.org/10.1007/978-3-030-19542-7_6

Students undoubtedly experience far more opportunities to observe a variety of interprofessional interactions in health care settings than they will ever have the chance to practice. This demands that the ability to learn from observation should be accorded a high priority in any course. It also implies that particular attention needs to be given to the role of simulations in promoting skills of observation as these are situations in which the role of observation can be directly influenced and acted upon, unlike the vicissitudes of opportunistic practice. However, developing skilled observation is not enough. Students need also to be able to respond to what they observe. At the very least they need to be able to formulate strategies to appropriately address the situations they identify, but they need also to be able to translate these plans into what is potentially actionable, and ultimately, act on them.

What are the circumstances that enable learning from observation in simulations? What kinds of observation practice can prompt students to develop the necessary capabilities? The major trap in simulation is to position observing students as passive and not engaged in the event. This is clearly not a desirable state of affairs as it is only through direct engagement and their own observations can they learn to discern what is important and identify what options they might have for dealing with expected and unexpected situations. While student observers may not, for example, be engaged in the hot action around the simulated patient, they can, if the overall event is set up appropriately, be just as actively engaged in noticing the action and recording what they see. They can practice their observation and be guided with respect to it through briefing and debriefing just as much as the players can be coached on their actions.

What then are the material conditions required and the set-up processes needed for observing practice to be fostered? The examples in this section show how easy it is to avoid observing the very phenomena that should be the focus of attention (interprofessional interactions) and for simulation processes to distract from the very learning that might be had. There is a predisposition in observing events of which one is not part, for following that which is most interesting and making premature judgements of what is occurring. While both seeing key actions and judging their appropriateness have a place, the challenge is to avoid them dominating initial exposure and for observers to miss out on noticing those things which might not be most exciting, but which contribute most to what they should be considering and thus learning.

These examples challenge us to look at the practices of simulation that enable and inhibit a focus on noticing and the consequences that flow from this. Adapting the practices of briefing, action and debriefing to fully accommodate the fact that observers should be as much part of the simulation as players is a necessary feature of the use of simulations for professional learning. After all, observers will inevitably become players and players will need to become sophisticated observers on many other occasions.

6.2   Learning Through Observation

Sofia Nyström · Madeleine Abrandt Dahlgren · Johanna Dahlberg
Linköping University
Linköping, Sweden
e-mail: sofia.nystrom@liu.se; madeleine.abrandt.dahlgren@liu.se;
johanna.dahlberg@liu.se

Organising simulation activities with large numbers of student brings on logistical challenges as well as consequences for what learning possibilities that become available, when some students are assigned to 'learning by doing' through participating actively in the scenario, and others to 'learning by observation' by watching the scenario being enacted by their peers. The fact that many students become observers of (simulated) clinical practice, rather than learning from first-hand experience of the future professional situation, raises pedagogical challenges. However, a vast majority of research on simulation focus on the learning of the acting students (Rochester et al. 2012). In this subsection, we will focus particularly on the conditions for learning from the simulation observers' point of view.

Previous research on learning from observation, or vicarious learning encompass learning contexts that include learning from observing someone else learn and learning from observing someone else act or perform (Chi et al. 2008). Studies on the value of observation for professional learning have been reported in various work settings (e.g. Köpsén and Nyström 2014). Focusing on education in healthcare, especially simulation-based education, some studies emphasise that not only physical and practical skills but also interprofessional and collaborative skills can be learned through vicarious learning (Chi et al. 2008; Grierson et al. 2012; Stegmann et al. 2012). However, Eikland Husebø et al. (2012) found that observing the training of other teams did not increase subsequent performance. When learning skills through simulation, a study by LeFlore et al. (2007) shows the value of observing instructors modelling ideal performance prior to students' own simulation experience. Another study (Stegmann et al. 2012) indicates that observing students learned as much as their peers, in doctor-patient communication skills, by observing their peers interact with standardised patents.

The conclusion the previous research is that learning by observing others is a complex issue especially when it comes to collaboration and team training. In this book, we apply an alternative approach to understand learning, where we ask how the practice of observation is arranged in simulation training and how it relates to the social and material arrangement of the simulation. The contexts in our studies are two different sites of undergraduate education of health professionals. The empirical data is based on video recordings and observational field notes of nursing and medical students engaged in simulations as a compulsory part of their education in the last semester before graduation (Nyström et al. 2016). Based on our findings, we will show how the material set-up and organisation of the observation create different learning conditions for the observing students. These different learning conditions are paramount for educators to understand in order to develop simulation activities that support the observing students learning.

6.2.1 Briefing: The Invitation to Participate as Observer

One key aspect of learning is how a task is introduced and thereby what expectations the instructors have on observers' participation. In line with previous research and as discussed Sect. 4.3, the briefing often focuses on the task of acting students and the simulation as such. However, research stresses the importance of engaging all students through a defined task justifying their role and giving value to their participation (O'Regan et al. 2016, p.10). In the context of our study, attention was generally redirected toward observers at the end of the briefing session. We noted a variety of ways in how the observing students were invited to engage in the forthcoming simulation (Nyström et al. 2016b). In some cases, the instructors justified the observer role and framed it as a learning situation.

> *Then, what about those of you that won't be in the simulation? Well, you will stay here in the observation room with the operator and me. What I say now is not my own words, but the students before you said that being an observer, watching what goes on and having a conversation with Theo and me, is not a waste of time. It is just another learning situation. You learn a lot from being observers, but it is different from being in there [points to the simulation room]. (Site 1- briefing 3)*

The observing students were also given specific tasks by the instructors, such as looking at communication and leadership. One instructor said "You will sit here and look for what the team performs well. It would also be good if you found one positive thing for each of your fellow students, and maybe one thing that could have been done differently."

We will now continue to discuss how these observations are thematised and made relevant for learning.

6.2.2 Observing Simulation

Our study had two different arrangements for the observing students. In one site, the students observed the simulation through a one-way screen, sitting together with the instructor and the operator in the control room (Nyström et al. 2016b). In the other site, the students were sitting in separate room, round at a table where they could watch the simulation on a screen. These two different socio-material arrangements had in common that the observing students had no possibility to change or interact with the simulation training that took place in front of them. This implies that the students' attunement was restricted and somewhat passive in relation to the material surrounding them, i.e. more like students in a classroom then active participant in a professional practice. In the following, we will now discuss the two ways in which the observation was arranged, proximate observation and distant observation.

6.2.2.1 Proximate Observation

When students were localised to the control room, observation emerged in a complex material set-up where the students were participating as a backstage audience, watching the scene from the coulisse. Here students were seeing different practices, i.e. the simulation exercise representing the professional practice of a hospital, the extension of the manikins' mind and bodily reactions via a voice through a loudspeaker, and how these bodily reactions were manipulated in the control room. This complexity was made possible due to the students' presence in the same room as the instructor and the operator running the scenario, but also their access and closeness to how the manikin was enacted by their fellow students, visualised via how the patient/manikin was operated via computer screens and different monitors.

The observing students could see how the patients' voice was enacted through the instructor, speaking into the microphone, and how this information was perceived by the students in the simulation room, influencing what was said and done on the other side of the one-way screen (Nyström et al. 2016b).

Interestingly, the observing students also heard and witnessed how the instructor or operator answered the phone call from the simulation room, acting "as if" they were other professional actors in the hospital setting.

> The operator answers the phone call from the simulation room saying: "The switch board". The medical student from the simulation room "I'm looking for the anaesthetist on call.". The operator continues, "Yes one moment.". He looks at the instructor, who laughs and states, "The anaesthetist is occupied". The operator talks into the phone again "Hi, it is Karen, mid-wife. You are paging the anaesthetist on call, they are here but they are occupied in the delivery department. Is it something you want me to pass on?" (Site 1 – observation 1) (Nyström et al. 2016b)

The study showed that the presence of the observing students located in the control room, close to the instructor shaped as a teaching practice. The teaching practice that emerged in this context, showed how the students became passive while the instructor was taking on a didactic teacher's role, using the simulation as an educational example of correct and incorrect professional behaviour or performance, but also used the location to inquire about students' medical knowledge or their knowledge of protocol.

> The students, instructor and operator hear the students in the simulation looking for a pulse on the screen in the simulation room. The instructor points to her screen and says "No, that is not the pulse, what is it?" She turns and looks at the observing students. One of the medical student answers, "It is Mean Arterial Pressure." Instructor says enthusiastic "Exactly! There are many parameters, here you have the heart rate. You have to know what the numbers stand for". (Site 1 – observing 4)

We also observed how the instructor redirected students' attention to certain events helping the students to distinguish critical instances in the simulation (Nyström et al. 2016b).

> *Through the one-way window, the students, the instructor, and the operator watch the students examining the patient, who starts to vomit. The instructor points out "Did you see how they took their time to position themselves in order turn the patient? It is not uncommon that someone just pulls [the instructor shows a pulling manoeuvre with the arm] the patient to one side [the students turn their attention towards the instructor]. Now look, let's see how they reposition the patient." All of them turn their attention towards the one-way window again. (Site 1- observing 3)*

In line with previous research, we emphasise that the presence of the instructor needs to be supportive in this respect, since research has shown that they have an important role in directing students' attention toward critical issues and ideal professional performances (see also Grierson et al. 2012; LeFlore et al. 2007). In this example, with proximate observation, the complexity of the socio-material arrangements in the control room where different practices coalise call for the importance of directing and supporting the observing students' attention towards the overarching aim of the simulation.

6.2.2.2   Distant Observation

In the case of distant observation, it was enacted in another socio-material set-up, characterized by a disconnection from the behind the scenes working of the actual simulation practice (Nyström et al. 2016b). At this location, the observation was distant to where the simulation took place, leaving students with no first-hand contact with the enactment of healthcare work by their peers. To guide their observations, they only had the short instruction from the instructor in the briefing saying that they should observe what their peers did well and what could have been done differently. We argue that this location and its material set-up form another type of pedagogical activity compared to proximate observation. The simulation was presented to the observing students as a projection of an activity on a screen, taking place somewhere else and therefore distant in space. The need of focus on the screen in order to hear and see what was played out made communication between the students sparse. Instead the observing students were sitting quietly around the table.

> *Four students sit around the table watching intensively a screen showing four images, one close-up of the manikin's upper body, two images from two different angles showing the hospital bed with the patient and two nurse students acting, and finally the screen with all the patient data. On the screen, they see one nurse student interacting with the patient and the other is trying to get hold of a doctor, without any success. The observing students fidget and laugh shortly. One of the observing nurse students says: What happened to the doctor? Why isn't anyone coming? Another one answer: I do not think the doctor is supposed to come yet. The group laugh nervously and continue to watch the screen. (Site 2 – observation 4)*

It was noticeable that the observing students' utterances and body language appeared to occur as a reaction to what was being projected from the simulation or as physical expressions of unease or dissatisfaction, indicating that the observation was a rather passive and individual activity compared to proximate observation. In this setting, the students had no instructor who could assist and guide their observation and the communication between the students were sparse, making these students more of a passive audience.

6.2.3 Support for Active Observation and Interprofessional Learning?

This chapter has discussed how the ways the material set-up and organisation of the observation create different learning conditions for the observing students. Previous research has emphasised that observation is an activity that needs to be supported (Chi et al. 2008; Stegmann et al. 2012) in order to achieve professional learning (e.g. Grierson et al. 2012; LeFlore et al. 2007). The findings show that the observation room/operator room is a pedagogical site of learning with its own material set-up, making certain activities more likely to happen (Schatzki 2002). We have shown two emerging methods of observation, proximate observation and distant observation. Proximate observation emerged in a complex material set-up where the students were participating as a backstage audience, watching the scene from the coulisse, seeing different practices, i.e. the professional practice of a hospital, the simulation exercise, and the extension of the manikin's mind and bodily reactions through the operator. The complexity of the sociomaterial arrangements the observers find themselves in, call for the importance of directing the students' attention towards what overarching aim of the simulation is. Here the presence of the instructor needs to be supportive in this respect, and in line with previous research the findings show that they are directing students' attention towards critical issues and professional performances (see also Grierson et al. 2012; LeFlore et al. 2007).

The findings also showed distant observation enacted in a different sociomaterial setup, characterised by a disconnection from the simulation practice. Here, the actual location was distant from the location where the simulation took place, leaving students with no first-hand contact with the enactment of healthcare work by their peers. Instead, the observing students are left to watch simulated healthcare work projected on a screen almost as an audience. In this setting, the interactions between the students are also passive, but in this setting, students have no instructor who can assist them in directing their observation.. Here, the actual location was distant from the location where the simulation took place, leaving students with no first-hand contact with the enactment of healthcare work by their peers. Instead, the observing students are left to watch simulated healthcare work projected on a screen almost as an audience. In this setting, the interactions between the students are also passive, but in this setting, students have no instructor who can assist them in directing their observation.

The aim of the simulation-based exercises was to practice interprofessional collaboration. However, our findings show that the observing students and the instructor have focus on professional behaviour and medical procedures more than articulating interprofessional collaboration. This could be seen as conflicting with the given task in the briefing, i.e. to observe communication, leadership and good/less good professional performance of the team. Based on the findings presented in this chapter, it is possible to question what conditions are created for learning interprofessional collaboration through the organisation and arrangements of the simulation-based training, especially when some are appointed to do simulation and others are to be observers.

The learning conditions for the observers could have benefited from being supported by an observational script, in order to get a more active learning experience (i.e. Chi et al. 2008). Such an observational script could also direct students gaze toward interprofessional aspects of the simulation. Reeves et al. (2011) emphasise that interaction between the learners are recommended for achieving interprofessional competencies. If students are given a specific task, could this direct student's observations to interprofessional behaviour? If so, how should this task be designed? One aspect is how to design a script that directs the observations towards the overarching aim of the simulation exercise, to develop interprofessional competencies. In the two enactments we have described, the students were passively watching the scene unfold. In one case, the activities were sometimes complemented with remarks from the instructor, or, as in the second case, distant observation were enacted in a sociomaterial set-up characterized by a disconnection from the physical interactions of the simulation. By this we mean that the observing students were left to watch simulated healthcare work projected on a screen, and the interactions between the students were passive, not having an instructor who assisted in directing their attention. Others have shown how the use of observational scripts could contribute to focus students' attention towards critical aspects of the simulation and increased the accuracy of the feedback provided by the observers (Stegmann et al. 2012), both individually and collaboratively (Zottmann et al. 2006).

6.2.4   Conclusions

- The findings contribute to knowledge on the complexity of arranging an observational practice within a simulation-based exercise.
- The two emerging ways of observation, enacting proximate observation and distant observation, have different material arrangements creating different conditions for learning, as well as differences in knowings that were emphasised and expressed.
- The results emphasise the importance of further understanding of how to use the observation room as a learning environment and a pedagogical site.

References

Chi, M.T.H., Roy, M., Hausmann, R.G.M. (2008). Observing tutorial dialogues collaboratively: Insights about human tutoring effectiveness from vicarious learning. *Cognitive Science, 32*, 301–341.

Dieckmann, P., Molin Friis, S., Lippert, A., Østergaard, D. (2012). Goals, success factors, and barriers for simulation-based learning: A qualitative interview study in health care. *Simulation & Gaming, 43*(5), 627–647.

Eikland Husebø, S., Bjørshol, C., Rystedt, H., Friberg, F., Søreide, E. (2012). A comparative study of defibrillation and cardiopulmonary resuscitation performance during simulated cardiac arrest in nursing student teams. *Scandinavian Journal of Trauma, Resuscitation and Emergency Medicine*, 20(23).

Grierson, L.E.M., Barry, M., Kapralos, B., Carnahan, H., Dubrowski, A. (2012). The role of collaborative interactivity in the observational practice of clinical skills. *Medical Education, 46*, 409–416.

Harder, N., Ross, C.J.M., Paul, P. (2013). Student perspective of roles assignment in high-fidelity simulation: An ethnographic study. *Clinical Simulation in Nursing*. https://doi.org/10.1016/j.ecns.2012.09.003.

Köpsén, S., & Nyström, S. (2014). The practice of supervision for professional learning: The example of future forensic specialists. *Studies in Continuing Education, 37*(1), 30–46.

LeFlore, J. L., Anderson, M., Michael, J. L., Engle, W. D., Anderson, J. (2007). Comparison of self-directed learning versus instructor-modeled learning during a simulated clinical experience. *Simulation in Healthcare, 2*(3), 170–177.

Nyström, S., Dahlberg, J., Hult, H., & Abrandt Dahlgren, M. (2016). Observing of interprofessional collaboration in simulation: A socio-material approach. *Journal of Interprofessional Care, 30*(6), 710–716. https://doi.org/10.1080/13561820.2016.1203297

Reeves, S., Goldman, J., Gilbert, J., Tepper, J., Silver, I., Suter, E., & Zwarenstein, M. (2011). A scoping review to improve conceptual clarity of interprofessional interventions. *Journal of Interprofessional Care, 25*, 167–174. https://doi.org/10.3109/13561820.2010.529960

Rochester, S., Kelly, M., Disler, R., White, H., Forber, J. Matiuk, S. (2012). Providing simulation experiences of large cohorts of 1st year nursing students: Evaluating quality and impact. *Collegian, 19*(3), 117–125.

Schatzki, T. (2002). *The site of the social: A philosophical account of the constitution of social life and change.* University Park: Pennsylvania State University Press.

Stegmann, K., Pilz, F., Siebeck, M. Fischer, F. (2012). Vicarious learning during simulations: Is it more effective then hands-on training? *Medical Education, 46*, 1001–1008.

Zottmann, J., Dieckmann, P., Rall, M., Fischer, F. Tarasow, T. (2006). Fostering simulation-based learning in medical education with collaboration scripts. *Simulation in Healthcare, 1*(3), 193.

6.3   Developing Professional Noticing: Shifting the Logic of Observer Guides from Evaluating to Noticing

Donna Rooney
University of Technology
Sydney, Australia
e-mail: donna.rooney@uts.edu.au

Michelle Kelly
Curtin University
Perth, Australia
e-mail: michelle.kelly@curtin.edu.au

6.3.1   Introduction

Students might understand the principles of "closed loop communication" and/or "holistic care". They might understand, in principle, the significance of any number of symptoms that patients may manifest. But noticing these sorts of activities and/ or other phenomena unfolding in an episode of professional practice requires practise. Most would agree, nursing and other health professions students need to become skilled in noticing multiple aspects within a range of complex clinical situations. This is both an issue for professional practice as much as it an issue for educators.

> Students need help recognizing the practical manifestations of textbook signs and symptoms, seeing and recognizing qualitative changes, in particular patient conditions, and learning qualitative distinctions among a range of possible manifestations, common meanings, and experiences. (Tanner 2006, p. 209)

According to Tanner's (2006) well-cited clinical judgement model (CJM), *noticing* is an essential step for nurses before they can interpret and respond to clinical situations – and a "function of nurses" expectations of the situation" (p. 208). But, if noticing is as "integral to the everyday practice of nurses" as Tanner and others suggest it is (Watson and Rebair 2014, p.154), then questions arise about how student nurses develop a capacity for noticing, in addition to questions about the sorts of pedagogical interventions which might promote it. Notwithstanding clinical placements and despite the limits of manikins (seen in Chap. 4), some may suggest that simulation-based education (SBE) provides a tentative answer to both questions. Promoting noticing behaviours, that is, helping novices to look and think beyond the obvious cues as they approach a patient or come across a "situation", can be afforded in SBE.

But what about students who observe simulation? Simulation based education (SBE) is fast becoming a "signature pedagogy" (Shulman 2005) of contemporary nursing education (and health education more broadly) that is informed by a mature research foundation including well-cited models of simulation in health education (e.g. Cook et al. 2011; Dieckmann et al. 2012). However, there is comparatively less available research that focuses attention on the large number of students taking observing roles (e.g. Grierson et al. 2012). Given increased enrolments, larger and diverse cohorts, limited practicum places, and diminishing resources among other things (Rochester et al. 2012), it seems timely to foreground the role of student observers in simulation classes.

This section begins with an overview of the observer role in simulation before turning specifically to noticing. Drawing on seminal ideas within health education literature (e.g. Tanner 2006; Lasater 2007), we introduce the concept of noticing, the first of four aspects in Tanner's research-based model, as central to making clinical judgements. Next, we briefly outline a two-phased Australian study where the observer role first captured our attention. We illustrate how the observers were prompted to *evaluate* the performance of their peers and consider this in terms of noticing. After offering an understanding of noticing that extends that found in the simulation literature, we move to the second phase of our study where we carried out a small pilot involving a series of interventions in an effort to make the observer experience a more active one. These interventions included the redevelopment of observer guides, that purposefully shift the logic of prompts from *evaluating* to *noticing* various aspects of the simulation and we illustrate how these generated more nuanced responses from observing students. We conclude by proposing multiple benefits of shifting the logic of observer guides, benefits in, and beyond, the simulation classroom.

6.3.2 The Observer Role

There are mixed views among students concerning being delegated an observer role. While some students prefer an observer role because it is perceived to be "less stressful" (Hober and Bonnel 2014; Kelly et al. 2016), others associate being an observer with "being bored" (Harder et al. 2013) and would prefer an acting role. Then there are roles like the documentation nurse, where the acting students come in and out of the action: offering a pseudo-observer experience, *with* opportunity to observe (closer to the action). Some students in Harder et al.'s study (2013) reported these betwixt roles as preferential. Regardless of students' perceptions and preferences for various roles in the simulation, studies concerned with learning highlight benefits of being an observer (O'Regan et al. 2016). These include: opening up thinking and analysis, engaging in the action via peer review, seeing the "bigger picture", validating one's own and others' practices and decisions, and, having a connection with the acting students in the simulation (Hober and Bonnel 2014).

An active/passive binary is often used to distinguish the acting role (active) from the observer role (passive) in simulation: with the former generally being more prized. The use of observation guides (sometimes called scripts or rubrics) by observers exemplifies a pedagogic intervention that seeks to make the observer role a more active one (Bethards 2014; Zottmann et al. 2018; Stegmann et al. 2012; Chi et al. 2008). These provide direction about *what* is to be observed (Bethards 2014). For instance, an observer guide may direct attention to various features of the simulation like clinical skills, teamwork or communication with an associated expectation that these will be learned, critiqued and promoted. There is much agreement that observer guides provide focus and structure to the observer role, and help observers contribute to more meaningful debriefings discussions (Bethards 2014; Stegmann et al. 2012; Zottmann et al. 2006; Chi et al. 2008). These sorts of findings led Stegmann et al. (2012) and others (e.g. Jeffries and Rizzolo 2006, in Scherer 2016, p.350) to conclude that learning experiences in simulation are equitable irrespective of learner role (see also Zottmann et al. 2018). Leaving the idea of 'equitable experiences' aside for the moment, given the importance of Tanner's CJM in nursing education, guides that focus observers' efforts on noticing, interpreting and reflecting are well regarded (e.g. Hober & Bonnel 2014).

6.3.3   Noticing in Clinical Judgement

Noticing is critical in all professional domains (Stürmer et al. 2015; Mason 2002). Teachers notice students' behaviour in their classrooms (Borich 2016), managers notice risks that need averting (Kutsch and Hall 2014), business leaders notice salient features of the market (Bazerman 2014) and nurses notice the clinical situations they are faced with. Tanner (2006) describes noticing as "[a] perceptual grasp of the situation at hand" (p. 208) and a first important step in making the clinical judgements which are central to the practice of nursing. Despite Tanner's (2006) CJM being over a decade old, it continues to inform research accounts of nursing and nurse education.

The CJM forms the basis of the Lasater Clinical Judgment Rubric (LCJR) (Lasater 2007). While the LCJR was designed to be used by educators to assess students' capacity for clinical judgement, it is telling to read how noticing is understood. First, the LCJR outlines examples of three dimensions of noticing: (1) focused observation; (2) recognizing deviations from expected patterns; and, (3) information seeking. Then, for each dimension, it provides criterion along a "beginning" through to "exemplary" continuum.

Beginning noticing involves:

1. Focused observation: important data [being] missed
2. Recognising deviation from expected patterns: focus[ing] on one thing at a time and miss[ing] most patterns and deviations
3. Information seeking: rely[ing] mostly on objective data (Lasater 2007 p. 500)

Whereas, *exemplary* noticing involves:

1. Focused observation: monitor[ing] a wide range of objective and subjective data
2. Recognising deviation from expected patterns: recogniz[ing] subtle patterns and deviations from expected patterns in data
3. Information seeking: carefully collect[ing] useful subjective data (Lasater 2007 p. 500)

6.3.4   Our Research and Subsequent Research Developments

Our interest in noticing is informed by insights into the observing role that emerged as part of a research study. Our initial aim was to conceptualize simulation in higher education. As our research progressed, a number of issues emerged in regard to observers of simulation (see Rooney et al. 2015; Kelly et al. 2016: Hopwood et al. 2014) and these became increasingly difficult to ignore. Each class consisted of around 25–30 students of which 5–7 were delegated an active role in each simulation, and the remaining (and majority) of the students were delegated observer roles. During the actual simulation, it was common to see observers engaged in personal grooming or playing with their mobile phones, and (in one instance) we even saw a student sleeping while the simulation was being performed. Despite all students having electronic access to observer guides prior to the class, only once was an observer guide actually seen (and this was left untouched on the student desk). When it came to the debriefing, it was typical for only one to three observers to contribute to discussions. In all, despite Stegmann et al.'s (2012) assertion that acting, and observers' roles were equitable, our general "hunch" was that the observers' experiences of simulation we saw during data collection were being overshadowed by the simulation action. We began to consider how the observer role and guides were introduced (or not) and what influence this might have on what observers did during the simulation.

Toward the end of our initial research an unanticipated opportunity arose to extend our study through a small internal "teaching and learning" grant. We used this as an opportunity to turn our attention to simulation observers and to pilot a number of interventions. We tried some changes to how student observers were organised including arranging them into small groups that each focused on a different aspect of the simulation. The results of this are described more fully elsewhere (Kelly et al. 2016). We made changes to facilitators' guides that included emphasising the value of observing (with a view to help students form intent for learning). We also identified how some facilitators were already prompting students to notice through "noticing out aloud" during the simulation (Rooney and Boud 2019).

But of particular interest here, is our redevelopment of the observer guides. With our focus on noticing, we rewrote observer guides and piloted them with four simulation cycles in the same subject as we had studied in the first phase of our research (e.g. Hopwood et al. 2014; Kelly et al. 2016; Rooney et al. 2015). Identical data collection processes to those used in the original research enabled us to comment on the outcomes of our developments. With an amendment to our original ethics approval, we also collected completed observer guides. The overall effect of these interventions resulted in major differences in observers' behaviour during the simulation and, as one observer attests, the students thought there were differences too:

> It was so good to actually have … normally the observers observe, and you'll talk about it at the end…but you might not really observe – having a focus area – you sit, and you think I actually have to work (laughs) it's really good to have the focus (class agree).

6.3.5 Evaluating Simulation

So, how was noticing (so critical to clinical judgement) reflected in the original (and generally unused) observer guides before our interventions? Well, the original observer guides prompted observers to notice *accomplished* simulated practice with questions like, "What elements of patient care did the team perform well?" An ideal response to this question involves observers noticing an isolated activity performed by their acting peers that they perceive as being performed in an *accomplished* manner. To evaluate it as such, they would need to compare their peers' performance with what they have learned about in class or from their textbooks.

It is not just our own institution that ask these sorts of questions. Zottmann et al.'s (2018) observation guide also prompts pairs of observers to find an "example of *successful implementation* of [effective communication]" (p. 4, *italics* in original). The directions are clear – not any example will do. Like our own prompts it must be an *accomplished* one and, like our own example, this form of questioning illustrates a logic of evaluation. Observers must focus on (notice) an activity and consider it in normative terms: i.e. how well the practice meets a shared understanding of normalised practice (Hopwood 2017, p. 70). Importantly, because it is an isolated activity that observers are prompted to notice/evaluate, it aligns with the LCJR beginning criterion of 'focusing on one thing at a time' in doing so the students' efforts could be assessed at a "beginning" level of noticing (Lasater 2007, p. 500). To be assessed more toward an "exemplary" level of noticing the prompts would need to guide observers to notice multiple activities; see/recognise patterns; and make judgements about subjective activities.

A similar framing is evident with another common prompt used in observer guides (or spoken during briefing sessions (see example in Sect. 6.2). This is where observers are asked to look for examples of their peers' acting performances that *do not* meet the shared understanding of accomplished practice. This sort of question also requires an understanding of what accomplished practice is, in order to consider why what their peers did was not. Again, this invites evaluative comments of an isolated activity that observers have noticed - again, according to Lasater's continuum, observers may be assessed at a "beginning level" of noticing (Lasater 2007, p. 500).

Another noteworthy point in regard to questions framed in this way is their purpose: i.e. to provide feedback to the acting students during debriefing sessions (Zottmann et al. 2018). In our institution's existing facilitator guides (based on commonly used formats), instructors were prompted to invite observers to provide feedback to their peers about their performances. While there is merit in peer feedback (Tai et al. 2017), and noticing/evaluating isolated examples of accomplished performances, these sorts of questions commonly found in observation guides may not be promoting a capacity for noticing as well as they could be. We suggest there are other forms of noticing that might complement and extend noticing – *and* to multiple ends. We stress, however, that we are not suggesting a replacement of the well-researched models of clinical judgement (if ever we could) but are suggesting a different perspective that encompasses and extends *what* and *how* observers of simulation might notice.

6.4   Expanding Noticing

By using the term noticing we mean more than simply seeing or 'becoming aware of' something (Dictionary.com). Indeed, elsewhere we propose three interrelated forms of noticing of relevance to SBE (Rooney and Boud 2019). The first form is *noticing in context*. Obviously pre-service nurse education must involve students learning the various activities that constitute nursing practice (e.g. taking blood pressure, performing CPR, patient handovers etc.). However, noticing in context refers to students understanding how the scope of activities that they are learning about unfold in a professional setting: not isolated enactments of a single activity. While well-rehearsed protocols (e.g. ABCDs etc.) do some work to illustrate how various activities hang together (e.g. airway, then breathing, then …), they do not account for episodes of professional practice when other activities (e.g. panicked family members, misplaced equipment, poor communication etc.) disrupt linear and non-situated sequences. To notice in this sense, is to be attuned to the spatial-temporal. Importantly, noticing in context requires noticing "more than one thing at a time" as well as the "subjective data" of a professional practice setting. In this way, noticing in context can foster "exemplary noticing" (Lasater 2007, p. 500).

Building on the first form of noticing, but also extending it, is *noticing of significance* (Rooney and Boud forthcoming). This second form of noticing refers to "disciplined perception" (Rose 2014, p.73) or "marking" (Mason 2002). For instance, within the professional setting, a nurse must not only notice when a patient's blood pressure has dropped but also recognise the significance of this. This is what Watson and Rebair (2014) refer to when they write of 'the art of noticing'. We understand noticing of significance in alignment to what Tanner (2006) advocates for in the CJM: i.e. being able to zoom in on and discern the salient features of clinical situations based on an understanding of what is likely to occur next – and what, if any, response is necessary. Noticing of significance also aligns with the concept of exemplary noticing through its invitation to recognize "deviations from expected patterns" (Lasater 2007, p. 500). Importantly, a capacity for noticing significance or 'marking' is dependent on the capacity to *notice in context*: This signals the interdependency of both forms of noticing presented hitherto.

Finally, as educators, we suggest that *noticing learning* itself constitutes a third, and necessary, form of noticing for simulation observers in pre-service professional education (Rooney and Boud 2019). As Bateson (1994) foreshadowed, the "essence of noticing is being awake to situations, being mindful rather than mindless" (in Mason 2002, p. 38). This means students forming an intent to learn prior to observing (Boud and Walker 1990) if they are to learn from it. While talking about experienced professionals ongoing professional learning, Billett (2016) also concurs that understanding one can learn by observing others, opens up the observing experience to learning. With an intent to learn from observing episodes of professional practice, students are able to notice (and reflect on) what was learned afterward as well. Like the other forms of noticing, we see *noticing learning* as important in pre-service education.

These three forms of noticing offer a different lens to consider the purposes and possibilities of observer guides used in simulation classes. For pre-service health professionals we see potential in working toward the exemplary levels of noticing that health practitioners require when making clinical judgements. However, we also see potential for developing skilled observers/noticers that may use their capacity for noticing to continue to learn as they enter their careers. Below we illustrate how we used these ideas to redevelop the observer guides used in a nursing subject in the second phase of our study.

6.4.1   From Evaluating to Noticing

In redeveloping the observer guides we expanded the evaluative logic of the original questions (described above) to include developing a capacity for noticing (see Table 6.1). The observers were divided into small groups that each had a different focus. Each group was given an observer guide with questions relating to their focus area. Some groups shadowed particular roles (e.g. team leader, nurse 1, patient etc.) and some groups focus was a particular phenomenon (e.g. communication, clinical actions etc.). In all the newly developed guides groups of observers were asked to notice specific actions or phenomena, and then expand on what they noticed in terms of impact/effect beyond quality. An ideal answer would not only indicate noticing a particular phenomenon but situating the activity in unfolding practice. For instance, observers shadowing the team leader were asked: "When does the TL step back from the action? What effect does this have?" To which, the observer group wrote: "The TL steps back when the TL calls the RMO for a drug order. When the TL steps back there was a bit of confusion". What we see here are students noticing in context: where "confusion" and the "team leader withdrawing" are temporarily linked in the unfolding practice being observed.

An example from another observation guide (with delegated focus on clinical actions) included asking: "What are the key clinical actions? How do these actions come about, and who instigates them?" A group responsible for this focus answered by stating: "Delivered Neb[ulizer].; Measurement shows patient has low Sat[uration]; RN1 decides to deliver nebulizer". In responding this way, the observers are *noticing* [the delivering a nebulizer] *in context* as well as *noticing* [the] *significance* of low oxygen saturation. Again, a temporal element links the occurrence of "low oxygen" with the "delivering nebulizer" in an unfolding sequence. The students were not only *noticing in context* but, according to Lasater (2007), demonstrating something more akin to exemplary noticing. Further questioning in the guide prompts observers

Table 6.1 Observer guide including questions and student responses

A. What are the clinical actions?	B. How do these actions come about, and who instigates them?	C. Does the action happen at the most appropriate time? Would it have been better at a different time?	D. What does this tell you about key ideas or concepts you already know about? What does this matter? What are the implications for your practice?
Clinical assessment	As soon as patient was admitted to the ED [emergency department], RN1 delegated roles (assessment)	Time management was well-managed. Patient seemed satisfied with the treatment he was receiving	Communicating with the patient is the essential factor in finding out patient's clinical problem
Change of NP [nasal prongs] – Hudson Mask	RN1 delegated the task to RN2 after the patient complains about SOB and chest tightness	Right time	Give immediate response to patient's complaints. Sharing nurses are here to care for you and building a good relationship between patient and nurses
The team gives/ administers pain relief	Asked how the patient was feeling – assessed their pain	Yes, it was appropriate because pain assessment was their first priority and they acted on it straight away	Listening to the patient – making sure they are comfortable

to notice and comment on the unfolding events *and* the timeliness of the action. To which another group responded: *"Patient was SOB* [short of breath] *and cough*[ing]. *Patient's symptoms were not resolved (intervention delivered not rapid enough)'* Here, students have not only noticed a temporal sequence (more than one thing), patterns and deviations (short breath, coughing, intervention), noticed the significance of symptoms (coughing short of breath), but also evaluated the temporality of what they had noticed. These rich examples of observers' noticing, via asking different sorts of questions, illustrates a shift toward exemplary noticing – consistent with the LCJR definitions (Lasater 2007, p.500).

Redeveloped guides were purposefully presented in a tabular format to illustrate the deliberate relationship between the questions. Below, for example, it is not just an isolated action (column A) that is to be noticed, but the guide prompts observers to notice its impact (column B) and timeliness (column C) as well. In addition, the fourth column (D) prompts students to think about (notice) what they are learning: this further extends the temporality of the simulation into their future practice.

Overall, these observation guides prompted students to engage with ideas and content that they already knew about, but in ways that extended what the earlier guides logic of evaluating practice had invited. These redeveloped guides include prompts for *noticing in context, noticing significance* and *noticing learning*. In terms of the continuum of noticing (Lasater 2007), they also shift the form of noticing from a beginning level through to developing, and towards accomplished and/or exemplary levels. In combination with other pedagogical strategies, like facilitator's briefing of observers and folding observers into debriefing sessions (Nyström, Abrandt Dahlgren and Dahlberg discuss this in more detail in Sect. 6.2), we mark this as a fruitful direction for further development and comments from observers' in our small trial provide additional encouragement:

> *I think the questions ...the observations questions thing ... is really good .... It.. so like X and I can sit here and say "do you think this is X" so we can discuss, and you can focus on the main points and then afterwards everyone can talk about it*

6.4.2   Noticing Beyond Simulation

Our small project of developing a pedagogy of noticing (in relation to observers of simulation) has potential to develop some capacity toward exemplary noticing as novice practitioners become involved in clinical judgement and actual clinical situations. However, here we point out additional benefits to developing a pedagogy of noticing. Supporting students to become more skilled observers (noticers) in the simulation classroom may develop a capacity for noticing that has other advantages as well. Throughout their careers our graduates will transition from novice to experienced practitioners and ongoing learning will be central to this. The combination of multiple opportunities to observe practice *and* being a skilled observer/noticer also presents ideal conditions for ongoing professional learning.

It is not only pre-service students in simulation classes that are observers. In professional settings it is common for novices and those on clinical placements to observe clinical situations. Billett (2016) goes further to explain how professionals engage in *mimetic* learning and how observing others in professional settings is central to this. Borrowing the Japanese term *minarai* (meaning apprentice) to make his point, he describes how learning through observation of professional practice is partially reliant on the learners' *intentionality* (Billett 2016 p.129). Observing, in this sense is an active process with an agentic element. In this sense, Billett aligns with early ideas about experiential learning: where, in order to learn from an experience, the learner must form some *intent* for learning (Boud and Walker 1996) – aligning with the broader intent of the activity itself (Hopwood 2017; Mahon et al. 2017). While we see helping observing students form learning intent as critical for educators in the simulation classroom, we also see value in helping students to independently recognise the potential for learning in practice situations long after they graduate. Perhaps what is needed is a reimagined fidelity that is pertinent to those who observe simulation as well as those who participate in acting roles – albeit in different ways?

6.5   Concluding Remarks

Simulation provides opportunities for developing capacity to *noticing context* as well as *noticing significance*. Observers of simulation can be assisted to 'read' the simulation action unfolding before them (*noticing in context*), notice significant features of it and predict what actions might be required (*noticing significance*). Pedagogical interventions, like carefully considered observer guides and framing observing as a learning experience, starting in the pre-briefing phase, can help students form learning intent (*noticing learning*). These are not alternatives to well-established research-based models currently used in nursing and health related pre-service education but complement and expand on the overall project of clinical judgement. Developing a 'pedagogy of noticing' in relation to patient cues, how teams communicate and respond to changing situations, may be a first step in guiding novice professionals to become skilled observers/noticers in other situations. The small intervention illustrated in this chapter shows that shifting the logic of observer guides has potential to also shift *what* and *how* observers of simulation are noticing and potentially moving them more toward the sorts of noticing required for patient care in professional practice. We mark this as a fruitful direction for further research.

- The logic of the prompts or questions in observer guides evoke different sorts of thinking and responses.
- Noticing in context, noticing significance and noticing learning build on and extend the forms of noticing that are prevalent in the health education literature (e.g. noticing in clinical judgement)
- Questions in observation guides that promote various forms of noticing can contribute to development of skilled observers/noticers
- Helping students develop a capacity for noticing may benefit them in, and beyond, the simulation classroom.

References

Bazerman, M. (2014) *The power of noticing: What the best leaders see.* New York: Simon & Schuster.

Bethards, M. (2014). Applying social learning theory to the observer role in simulation. *Clinical Simulation in Nursing, 10*(2), e65–e69. https://doi.org/10.1016/j.ecns.2013.08.002.

Billett, S. (2016). Learning through health care work: Premises, contributions and practices. *Medical Education, 50*, 124–131. https://doi.org/10.1111/medu.12848.

Borich, G. (2016). *Observation skills for effective teaching: Research-based practice* (7th ed.). New York: Routledge.

Boud, D., & Walker, D. (1990). *Learning from experience: Using experience for learning.* Buckingham: Open University Press.

Chi, M. T. H., Roy, M., Hausmann, R.G.M. (2008). Observing tutorial dialogues collaboratively: Insights about human tutoring effectiveness from vicarious learning. *Cognitive Science, 32*, 301–341. https://doi.org/10.1080/03640210701863396.

Cook, D.A., Hatala, R., Brydges, R., Zendejas, B., Szostek, J.H., Wang, A.T., et al. (2011). Technology-enhanced simulation for health professions education: a systematic review and meta-analysis. *JAMA. 306*(9), 978–88. https://doi.org/10.1001/jama.2011.1234.

Dieckmann, P., Molin Friis, S., Lippert, A., Østergaard, D. (2012). Goals, success factors, and barriers for simulation-based learning: a qualitative interview study in health care. *Simulation & Gaming, 43*(5), 627–647. https://doi.org/10.1177/1046878112439649.

Grierson, L.E.M., Barry, M., Kapralos, B., Carnahan, H., Dubrowski, A. (2012). The role of collaborative interactivity in the observational practice of clinical skills. *MedicalEducation,46*,409–416.https://doi.org/10.1111/j.1365-2923.2011.04196.x.

Harder, N., Ross, C. J., Paul, P. (2013). Student perspective of roles assignment in high-fidelity simulation: An ethnographic study. *Clinical Simulation in Nursing, 9*(9), e329–e334. https://doi.org/10.1016/j.ecns.2012.09.003.

Hober, C., & Bonnel, W. (2014). Student Perceptions of the observer role in high-fidelity simulation. *Clinical Simulation in Nursing, 10*(10), 507–514. http://dx.doi.org.ezproxy.lib.uts.edu.au/10.1016/j.ecns.2014.07.008

Hopwood, N. (2017). Practice architectures of simulation pedagogy: from fidelity to transformation. In K. Mahon, J. Kaakinen, S. Francisco, S. Kemmis & A. Lloyd (Eds.), *Exploring educational and professional practice: Through the lens of practice architectures* (pp. 63–82). Singapore: Springer.

Hopwood, N., Rooney, D., Boud, D., & Kelly, M. (2014). Sociomateriality, simulation and methods. Second International ProPEL conference "Professional Matters: Materialities and Virtualities of Professional Learning", Stirling, United Kingdom.

Kelly, M.A., Hopwood, N., Rooney, D., & Boud, D. (2016). Enhancing students' learning through simulation: Dealing with diverse, large cohorts. *Clinical Simulation in Nursing, 12*(5), 171–176. https://doi.org/10.1016/j.ecns.2016.01.010.

Kutsch, E. & Hall, M. (2016). *Project Resilience: The art of noticing, interpreting, preparing, containing and recovering*. London: Routledge.

Lasater, K. (2007). Clinical judgement development: Using simulation to create an assessment rubric. *Journal of Nursing Education, 46*(11), 496–503.

Mahon, K., Kemmis, S., Francisco, S., & Lloyd, A. (2017). Introduction: practice theory and the theory of practice architectures. In K. Mahon, J. Kaakinen, S. Francisco, S. Kemmis & A. Lloyd (Eds.), *Exploring educational and professional practice: Through the lens of practice architectures* (pp. 1–30). Singapore: Springer.

Mason, J. (2002) *Researching your own practice: The discipline of noticing.* London: Routledge Falmer.

O'Regan, S., Molloy, E., Watterson, L., Nestel, D. (2016). Observer roles that optimise learning in healthcare simulation education: A systematic review. *Advances in Simulation, 1*(1). https://doi.org/10.1186/s41077-015-0004-8.

Rochester, S., Kelly, M., Disler, R., White, H., Forber, J., Matiuk, S. (2012). Providing simulation experiences of large cohorts of 1st year nursing students: evaluating quality and impact. *Collegian, 19*(3), 117–125. https://doi.org/10.1016/j.colegn.2012.05.004.

Rooney, D., & Boud, D. (2019). *Toward a pedagogy for professional noticing: Learning through observation. Vocations and Learning.* 1–17. https://doi.org/10.1007/s12186-019-09222-3.

Rooney, D., Hopwood, N., Boud, D., Kelly, M. (2015). The role of simulation in pedagogies of professional formation: A practice theory view in the higher education context. *Vocations and Learning.* https://doi.org/10.1007/s12186-015-9138-z.

Rose, M. (2014). *The mind at work: Valuing the intelligence of the American worker* (2nd ed.). New York: Penguin Books.

Scherer, Y., Foltz-Ramos, K., Fabry, D., Chau, Y. C. (2016). Evaluating simulation methodologies to determine best strategies to maximize student learning. *Journal of Professional Nursing, 32*(5), 349–357. https://doi.org/10.1016/j.profnurs.2016.01.003.

Shulman, L. (2005). Signature pedagogies in the professions. *Daedalus, 134*(3), 52–59.

Stegmann, K., Pilz, F., Siebeck, M., Fischer, F. (2012). Vicarious learning during simulations: Is it more effective than hands-on training. *Medical Education, 46,* 1001–1008. https://doi.org/10.1111/j.1365-2923.2012.04344.x.

Stürmer, K., Könings, K. D., Seidel, T. (2015). Factors within university-based teacher education relating to preservice teachers' professional vision. *Vocations and Learning, 8*(1), 35–54. https://doi.org/10.1007/s12186-014-9122-z.

Tai, J., Ajjawi, R., Boud, D., Dawson, P., Pandaero, E. (2017). Developing evaluative judgement: Enabling students to make decisions about the quality of work. *Higher Education, 76,* 467–481. doi.org/10.1007/s10734-017-0220-3.

Tanner, C. (2006). Thinking like a nurse: A researched-based model of clinical judgment in nursing. *Journal of Nursing Education, 45*(6), 204–211.

Watson, F., & Rebair, A. (2014). The art of noticing: Essential nursing practice. *British Journal of Nursing, 23*(10), 514–517. https://doi.org/10.12968/bjon.2014.23.10.514.

Zottmann, J., Dieckmann, P., Taraszow, T., Rall, M., F, F. (2018). Just watching is not enough: Fostering simulation-based learning with collaboration scripts. *GMS Journal for Medical Education, 35*(3), 1–18. https://doi.org/10.3205/zma001181.

6.6 Commentary

Dara O'Keeffe
Royal College of Surgeons in Ireland
Dublin, Ireland
e-mail: daraokeeffe@rcsi.ie

This chapter has discussed the role of the observers of simulation from two contexts. Firstly, how the setup of the observation environment affects learning; and secondly how the learner's observation skills can be enhanced.

The structure or setup of the observation environment is a fascinating issue. The authors here describe two potential environments: proximate and distant. Proximate observation is defined here as observing from the control room with running commentary from the instructor. In this setup there is proximate feedback from the instructor however, the observers being in the control room breaks the high fidelity of the simulation, bringing their frame of mind away from a believable clinical context and showing the activity from a very different viewpoint. It may be hard for observers in this situation to project themselves into the frame of mind of someone immersed in the scenario and they may therefore not be able to understand why the performing learners have carried out certain actions.

Distant observation is described here as locating the learners in an observation room without a facilitator present and it has been shown that this leads to a more "passive" learning environment. This kind of environment will undoubtedly be less effective unless it is actively setup by introducing tasks to the learner in advance via what is described here as an 'Observation script' (Bethards 2014; Stegmann et al. 2012; Zottmann et al. 2006; Chi et al. 2006). However, this alone may not produce the desired effect in learning. Giving defined observation tasks in advance should also include a clear outline of the learning objectives for the learners, as without this they may focus on the wrong outcomes, for example, assessing the individuals' performance instead of the inter-professional interactions.

We pose the question as to whether the difference between these two environments is really the location, but actually more about the presence or absence of a facilitator to give proximate feedback? We would suggest that there is a third observation setup environment that will compensate for the disadvantages of both these previously described situations. That setup involves proximate feedback being given by a facilitator from a remote or adjacent observation room without the distraction of the control room environment. This setup requires additional faculty but probably yields the best observational learning experience for the observers.

In the second part, learners' observation skills are discussed in the context of shifting focus from "Evaluating" to "Noticing" behaviours and performance. Traditional observation guides tend to focus on objective evaluation of tasks performed but the authors here discuss how framing these guides to encourage more advanced 'noticing' encourages pattern recognition and other higher-level observation skills. In our institution, we promote this in the observers by asking them in advance what they hope to observe (after they have heard the case presentation) and how they will "notice" if this has been achieved. This concept of advanced noticing is then reinforced during our instructor debriefing which uses the Advocacy Inquiry approach (Rudolph et al. 2008) in which the facilitator will repeatedly model the "I noticed" framework and language, thereby reinforcing the noticing behaviours from the learners. The 'noticing of significance' described above is also reinforced by this framework by indicating why the behaviour caused concern for the instructor. This is just one example of how advanced noticing can be promoted both before and after the simulation is observed. The authors make the important point that teaching higher level noticing and evaluating skills in simulation may well translate to improvement of these skills in the clinical environment.

Logistical issues can sometimes impact negatively on instructors attempts to provide equity of experience between participants and observers. Very large class groups where only a small number of learners will participate in the simulation and the majority remain as observers provides a huge challenge to equity of learning. High fidelity simulation was not originally conceived to be used in large groups. However, enthusiasm for simulation as a mode of teaching implementation has led to increased pressure on educators to use simulation in learning contexts that are not ideally suited to this modality. How much time do we realistically have as instructors to teach the observers to observe? Sometimes we must accept that this learning will happen longitudinally over years as they advance through their training experiencing repeated simulation sessions.

Being mindful of supporting the correct pedagogy and providing the correct structure to the observation environment should lead to an equitable learning experience for participants and observers alike as discussed above (Jefferies and Rizzolo 2006; Zottmann et al. 2018). However, to ensure optimum equity in learning we need to consider the structure of the simulation session as a whole and plan to allow all learners to be both participant and observer during multiple simulations wherever possible. This will ensure the most holistic learning experience for all participants in the simulated environment.

Reference

Rudolph, J., Simon, R., Raemer, D., & Eppich, W. (2008). Debriefing as formative assessment: Closing performance gaps in medical education. *Academic Emergency Medicine, 15*, 1010–1016.

Chapter 7
Reflecting on Interprofessional Simulation

Sissel Eikeland Husebø, Madeleine Abrandt Dahlgren, Samuel Edelbring, Elin Nordenström, Torben Nordahl Amorøe, Hans Rystedt, and Peter Dieckmann

7.1 Introduction

Sissel Eikeland Husebø
University of Stavanger
Stavanger, Norway
e-mail: sissel.i.husebo@uis.no

The debriefing is a crucial aspect of interprofessional simulation-based education in healthcare. The debriefing phase is an activity that follows a simulation experience and are usually led by a facilitator. The debriefing aims to encourage participants'

S. E. Husebø
University of Stavanger, Stavanger, Norway
e-mail: sissel.i.husebo@uis.no

M. Abrandt Dahlgren (✉)
Linköping University, Linköping, Sweden
e-mail: madeleine.abrandt.dahlgren@liu.se

S. Edelbring
Örebro University, Örebro, Sweden
e-mail: samuel.edelbring@oru.se

E. Nordenström · T. Nordahl Amorøe · H. Rystedt
University of Gothenburg, Gothenburg, Sweden
e-mail: elin.nordenstrom@ped.gu.se; torben.nordahl-amoroe@vgregion.se;
hans.rystedt@ped.gu.se

P. Dieckmann
Copenhagen Academy for Medical Education and Simulation (CAMES),
Center for Human Resources, Capital Region of Denmark, Copenhagen, Denmark

Department for Clinical Medicine, University of Copenhagen, Copenhagen, Denmark

Department for Quality and Health Technology, University of Stavanger, Stavanger, Norway
e-mail: mail@peter-dieckmann.de

© Springer Nature Switzerland AG 2019   139
M. Abrandt Dahlgren et al. (eds.), *Interprofessional Simulation in Health Care*,
Professional and Practice-based Learning 26,
https://doi.org/10.1007/978-3-030-19542-7_7

reflective thinking and provide feedback about their performance, while various aspects of the completed simulation is discussed. Previous research on debriefing has focused mostly on how debriefing affects learning, behaviors, and patient outcomes, while few studies have investigated what is going on in the debriefing in order to better understand the complexity inherent in this phase of the simulation activity and how the practice of debriefing can support participants achieving the learning objectives.

The first section aims to give a short overview of how debriefing is described in the simulation literature, the use of practice-based, empirical research on debriefing in interprofessional simulation activities, and to discuss in what ways this kind of research contribute to the theorizing of simulation pedagogies. It also places emphasis on the many other critical aspects around the practicalities of debriefing, which are "the what, who, when, where, and how to debrief". Reflection on experience stands out as a general feature that needs to be addressed in order to achieve a successful debriefing for learning. Of notable importance is that the authors take a clear stand that debriefing is a practice, embedded in and interrelated, or bundled with social and material arrangements. The aim of the interprofessional simulation activity was to practice team collaboration. The authors base their analysis of video-recorded debriefing sessions, with nursing and medical students and with professional nurses and physicians. The findings show that emergent practices in interprofessional debriefing reveal similarities, but also some important differences between students and professionals, respectively. The similarities identified between the students and professionals' debriefings were related to instructions of thinking about, describing individual issues the participants did well and what they could improve. There was also similarity in the sense that the individual actions in the scenario risk overshadowing the objective of interprofessional collaboration, which is more seldom thematized in the debriefings of student and professional teams. The students were more concerned with the biomedical knowledge and the correctness in professional behavior associated with the sequence of events unfolding in the scenario than professionals were.

The second section aims to present and discuss how video can be used as a tool for feedback and reflection in debriefing to support interprofessional learning. The subsection is based on data from a series of one-day interprofessional training occasions for nursing and medical students. The objectives of the simulation sessions were to train methods of structured examination and communication. The analysis revealed that when the facilitators introduced a video-clip before it was shown in the debriefings, a model with "open-ended" and "specific" strategies were identified. An introduction with the "open-ended" strategy provided only brief information about the situation in the video clip and no instruction for what aspects to focus and reflect upon, while the "specific" strategy provided what actions to observe and the reasons for doing so. Since both strategies have pros and cons a model with more context dependent model was developed. The model suggests four interrelated aspects that should be taken into account when choosing which strategy to use when introducing video clips. The two examples presented in this section show that video clip provides a third-person perspective that can be used to re-conceptualize how participants' conduct is to be seen and assessed in relation to the demands of interprofessional teamwork. The video is central as a basis for discussion and reflections, but for inexperienced participants the instructors' guidance is critical for viewing the recorded events as relevant to teamwork.

7.2 Debriefing in Simulation-Based Education

Madeleine Abrandt Dahlgren
Linköping University
Linköping, Sweden
e-mail: madeleine.abrandt.dahlgren@liu.se

Samuel Edelbring
Örebro University
Örebro, Sweden
e-mail: samuel.edelbring@oru.se

Debriefing in simulation-based education is often emphasised as the most critical and important phase of simulation to support participants' learning (Dieckmann 2009; Raemer et al. 2011). In the debriefing, participants' emotional reactions, actions and interactions in the scenario are traditionally brought up as topics for reflection. Fanning and Gaba (2007) state that debriefing is one way to bridge the gap between experiencing an event and learning from it.

Historically, debriefing has its origin in the military and aviation domains as a means of following up on the people's experiences of participating in crisis situations. Debriefing makes possible an accounting of a mission and allows the participants to express and discuss emotions to mitigate their stress (Gough et al. 2012). Dreifuerst and Decker (2012) describe how debriefing has migrated to a variety of fields and propose that debriefing in health care serves three purposes: "…to receive an accounting, to mitigate emotional response, and to correct decisions and actions that were incorrectly applied in the simulation experience". The ideas of how to arrange and conduct simulation have migrated into health care from other areas than education. Medical simulation is thus influenced by military after-action review, simulation and procedures for safety in aviation, dating back to the early twentieth century (Singh et al. 2013). The migration of simulation into professional health care has brought about a tradition of the pedagogy for simulation activities following a predefined set of stages that has been labelled briefing, simulation and debriefing (e.g. Dieckmann 2009).

Simulation based education is often described as learner-centred approach because of reliance on learners' activity and active participation. Educational references are often inspired by i experiential learning theory, drawing on the work of Kolb and Dewey and involving multiple aspects of learning such as cognitive, affective and psycho-motor dimensions (Rooney et al. 2015). Rooney et al., however, suggest in their overview of the conceptual basis for simulation that although there is a mature body of research in simulation, the theoretical basis for simulation pedagogies is limited. The adequacy of the conceptual basis for simulation pedagogies has been questioned (e.g. Berragan 2011; Dieckmann et al. 2012; Poikela and Teräs 2015). Poikela and Teräs (2015) identified in their scoping review of learning in nursing simulation 13 different conceptualisations of learning in simulation-based education, often taking the concepts given for granted without explaining or exploring their theoretical and historical roots. Rooney et al. (2015, p. 273) argue that there is a need for a theoretical understanding that can provide directions for empirical research that answers to fundamental pedagogical questions as "why we use simulation in healthcare education and what it would mean for this to be done well' (see Chap. 1, this volume for further discussion). In this chapter, we will use practice-based, empirical research on debriefing and discuss in what ways this kind of research contribute to the theorizing of simulation pedagogies. Before we do this, we will make a short overview of how debriefing is described in the simulation literature.

7.2.1   What Goes on in Debriefing?

Jeffries (2013) describes debriefing as following is a multitude of debriefing models to meet different learning outcomes. A general feature of these models is that they prescribe a defined sequence of descriptive, analytic and application phases that the debriefing should follow (e.g. Steinwachs 1992; Rudolph et al. 2006). A structured model of debriefing has sometimes been referred to as comprising at least three phases "Reactions", "Understanding" and "Summarize" (Gardner 2013, Rudolph et al. 2006). Following a structured model has been claimed to provide clarity to the learners regarding the debriefing process and to facilitate better reflections (Neill and Wotton 2011). Reflection on experience stands out as a general feature that needs to be addressed in order to achieve a successful debriefing for learning. Dieckmann et al. (2012) argue that the participants need to reflect upon their experiences in order to reconstruct and transform their simulation experiences from into learning and practice. Other authors take the more radical position on reflection stating that reflection is not only helpful, but a requirement in order to at all learn from simulation experiences (Crookall 2014). In a critical review of debriefing methods, Sawyer et al. (2016) provide an overview of how the wide variety of debriefing methods available can be structurally categorized according to *timing, conversation facilitation, conversation structure and process elements*. The most common timing of the debriefing is generally *postevent*, i.e. takes place after the simulation is completed. This is also our focus in this chapter, and we will limit our discussion to post-event debriefing. Post-event debriefing is either facilitator-guided, i.e. structured and led by a facilitator and following a pre-defined conversational structure, or self-guided by the participants. The conversation structure within the debriefing conversation unfolds during facilitator-guided postevent debriefing in generally three (or more) phases where participants narrate, analyse and apply their experience (Sawyer et al. 2016). The narration phase includes in some, but not all, frameworks a 'reaction' phase in order to deal with reactions and/or emotions.

A description of how this guidance is conducted is described e.g. by Rudolph et al. (2008). In the first stage, Rudolph et al. (2008), argue that learners need to have the opportunity to "blow off steam". In the second phase the instructor directs awareness to the simulation activity in relation to learning objectives. While the instructor often suppresses evaluative comments in the reaction phase, it is common, according to Rudolph et al. (2008) both for participants and facilitator to use the analysis phase in an evaluative manner. In the summary phase participants consolidate lessons learned and typically express what they will carry forward from the experience.

Sawyer et al. (2016) identified common process elements across different debriefing models. These comprise essential elements such as e.g. ensuring psychological safety, clarifying basic assumptions, mental models and debriefing rules, addressing learning objectives and the use of open-ended questions. Among other conversational techniques/educational strategies identified were learner self-assessment and directive feedback. A further strategy was to use circular questions where a third party is invited to re-narrate the course of events involving two other participants of the team. Another technique was advocacy inquiry (where the facilitator shares her interpretation of what happened during a sequence of events and invites a participant to share his reasons for and understanding of what happened).

Other studies have suggested that the facilitator style, or dynamics of how the facilitator interacts with the participants in the debriefing phase may influence the process and outcome of the debriefing (Dieckmann et al. 2012). Previous research has also shown that it can be difficult to facilitate deep reflection with participants. Husebø et al. (2013) showed that the instructors' probing questions in the debriefing are often too descriptive in order to be productive. Kihlgren et al. (2015) adopted a previously developed framework for analyzing levels of reflection and applied the framework on utterances in 38 debriefing sessions with 10 instructors conducting the debriefing. The findings showed that the participants' reflections levels were usually low, and seemingly indifferent of the debriefers' utterances. There is a need, the authors argue, for future research on debriefing to develop a more analytical framework for probing questions in order to facilitate deeper reflection. Saywer et al. (2016) states that despite the volume of available literature on debriefing in health care simulation, there is limited evidence in support of a specific debriefing model (Cheng et al. 2014; Raemer et al. 2011). They suggest that it is very likely that there is no "best" way to conduct a debriefing, but that there are a variety of methods to choose from, depending on their respective context, and their own skill set and preferences.

7.2.2 Re-thinking Debriefing in Interprofessional Simulation

In this chapter, we apply a practice theory perspective on debriefing, and argue that there is a need to situate simulation-based education as a pedagogical arrangement in accordance with recent theorizations of professional knowledge and learning (see Chap. 2 for more details on practice theory). A practice theory approach means to move beyond the historical psychological roots of debriefing as part of reconciliation of a traumatic experience. It means to re-think debriefing as a practice, embedded in and interrelated, or bundled with social and material arrangements. The social (interaction, collaboration, hierarchies, etc.) are bundled with the material (setting, physical equipment, protocols, schedules, etc.). Prefiguration means in this sense, that arrangements make it more or less likely for participants to follow some paths than others (Schatzki 2012). A practice can thereby not be determined or designed in advance but unfolds through the sequence of actions. In following such a perspective, the traditional conceptual models for debriefing become insufficient to capture the full complexity of the evolving scenario. Rooney et al. (2015) argue that there is a need of including also the material arrangements into the analysis, i.e. the simulator and the material set-up for the simulation. These material arrangements are seen as active components of the practice, and therefore also potentially influence the learning outcome in ways that go beyond abstract outcome measures and experimental comparisons (Rooney et al. 2015).

In the following, we will look closer into debriefing of interprofessional simulation activities. We will base our analyses on empirical studies of simulation activities, with nursing and medical students at the final stages of their educational training (Nyström et al. 2016a), and with professional nurses and physicians, as they debrief interprofessional simulation (Nyström et al. 2017). While research on health professionals in simulation activities is quite common, reviews of research on interprofessional simulation-based training show that studies focusing on the practice of simulation in undergraduate programs, like the ones we refer to in this subsection, are sparse (Gough et al. 2012; Palaganas et al. 2014). Research in interprofessional education (IPE) and simulation in undergraduate training have predominantly concerned evaluation of courses, learners' perspective of IPE, and teamwork outcomes (Cook et al. 2011). Some studies also focused on the learners' attitudes and their learning about the roles and skills of other professions or disciplines (Gough et al. 2012; Alinier et al. 2014).

When it comes to simulation-based education in undergraduate health care programs, it can be argued that the learners in this context differ from professional practitioners, who participate in simulation as part of their continuing education in the workplace. The health professionals are there to practice skills that they have already gained in their previous training and are able to relate events to an everyday professional practice. To the health professionals, the acute situation is familiar, but occurs less often, and hence needs to be practiced and refreshed under safe conditions. The students, on the other hand are there to develop professional skills that they have not yet fully acquired, in a practice situation that might be new to them. In the following, we will show that emergent practices in interprofessional debriefing reveal similarities, but also some important differences between students and professionals, respectively. The differences in how the debriefing is enacted have some important implications for educators and practitioners who are involved in simulation training. In next section, we will compare the characteristics of the emerging interprofessional debriefing practices and discuss how the insights drawn from the research may inform design and facilitation of learning in these activities.

7.2.3 *Interprofessional Simulation Debriefing Practices:* *Students and Professionals*

The aim of the interprofessional simulation activities studied, both for students and for professionals, was to practice team collaboration in acute settings. For the students, the activity aimed at supporting learning related to intended interprofessional and common learning outcomes, as well as program specific intended learning outcomes for emergency care for the nursing and medical program respectively. Examples of common IPE objectives are interprofessional role taking, responsibilities and communication (Nyström et al. 2016b). The data we refer to in this section is based on video recordings from 18 debriefing sessions with medical and nursing students from two different sites of professional health care education (see Chap. 3 for a detailed description of how data were collected). We also draw on analyses of video-recordings from ten debriefing sessions from two different sites, where professional physicians and nurses participated in interprofessional simulation as a continuing professional development activity (Nyström et al. 2017).

Drawing on practice theory in our collaborative analyses of video-recorded debriefing sessions with nursing and medical students (see Chap. 2 for a detailed description of practice theory and Chap. 3 for a description of the collaborative analysis), we show how debriefing practices emerge following two distinctive patterns. These two patterns could be described as *algorithm* or as *laissez-faire*. The emerging patterns of debriefing practices were relational to material objects, such as the protocols and arrangements of the debriefing room, but also to intentions of collegiality. In our studies of video-recorded debriefing sessions with physicians and nurses, participating in simulation training as a continuing development activity, some resemblances with the debriefing sessions with students were identified, but also distinctive differences, the awareness of that we argue can be of value for designing interprofessional simulation training.

7.2.4 *Students' Debriefing as* Algorithm

Our findings show that how the students' doings, sayings and interactions during the simulation were invited as topics for discussion and reflection shapes the debriefing session differently. One of the patterns of students' debriefing identified, *algorithm,* could be described as a procedure following a certain protocol. The protocol is bundled with the debriefing practice in that it produces a pattern of interactions between the participants, which follows predefined steps as the debriefing unfolds. The protocol was enacted through the facilitator through a closed inquiry approach, which adhered closely to the pre-defined steps. The pre-defined steps introduce an agenda for what was legitimate to bring up for discussion and reflection (Nyström et al. 2016b).

The students, dressed in white clinical clothes, drop in after the simulation, sit down around the table and engage in small talk with each other. The instructor enters, dressed in everyday clothes, and all the students turn their attention towards him. The instructor starts: "So we are going to debrief now. We think it is a good idea that you do not discuss the scenario with each other beforehand because we believe that we should do it together here in the debriefing. We use a certain model for debriefing. Sometimes when you have done or experienced something you have a tendency to be self-critical and talk about what you could have done differently. We believe that it's not the best way to analyse this./.../ we usually say that we have three steps. First we talk about what happened, completely factual. Because it is not certain that we all saw what happened [during the scenario] and then we analyse. We do that by first talking about what we did well. We do that so we become aware what it is that I or we are good at, so we can continue doing that and then we can continue to maybe talk about what we could have done differently. And lastly, we also discuss how we can use this scenario, and we will also look a little at a video sequence. But before we get going I want to start by asking how you are feeling at the moment? Johan?" Johan, a nursing student, clears his throat and answers: "Confused... " (Field note 1: Site 2)

We can note here that the first step of the debriefing is introducing the rationale of the debriefing as avoiding self-criticism, starting with the individual and not immediately sharing experiences. The process and sequence of the debriefing is laid out as following three phases; step one comprising a descriptive, *"completely factual"* a neutral re-construction of the activities during the scenario. The second phase is introduced as the analysis phase, of which the first part should focus on affirmation – *"what went well and what we are good at"*. The third part of the analysis phase should focus of what could *"have been done differently"*. The final step of the debriefing is introduced as focusing what to take forward from the simulation exercise as implications for practice, *"how we can use this scenario"*, also including the watching of videoclips. When the sequence of the three phases is described, a fourth step focusing on the emotional reactions *"how you are feeling at the moment"* is introduced and make up the very start of the debriefing process.

7.2.5   Students' Debriefing as Laissez-faire

As a contrast to the *algorithm*, a second distinctive pattern of students' debriefing that can be described as *laissez-faire* was identified. If we compare this debriefing pattern to the *algorithm*, the *laissez-faire* can be described as a collegial conversation without an explicit pre-defined structure or expressed aims. The facilitator's sayings and doings have the characteristics of a chairperson – initiating the conversation and facilitating turn-taking. As shown below, this pattern acts on the debriefing practice differently, through the facilitator's sayings as an open inquiry approach.

The students, dressed in white clinical clothes, burst into the room after the simulation and try to grab a chair. You can hear a voice outside the room saying: "We will need more chairs in here." The students talk to each other and then the instructor, dressed in green clinical clothes, comes in and while she is trying to find a chair she says: "OK, good folks. So, let's have free comments from all of you, actors as well as those who observed!" And then she leans back in her chair. One of the medical students starts immediately and says: "Well I still haven't phoned the doctor on call. I, it is hard to remember to phone the doctor on call. I just, oh yes the doctor on call." And she and the other students as well as the instructor laugh a bit and the instructor says: "Well absolutely, it could have been a good idea, but it went well anyway. Somebody else? " (Field note 4: Site 1)

We can note here how the introduction of the debriefing process is organised as an open invitation for free comments to all participants. There are no instructions for how the reflections should be structured or in what order what kind of reflections should be addressed. The *laissez-faire* pattern of debriefing prefigured the reflection participant-driven and loosely structured around the sequence of activities and interactions during the simulation. There were no protocols or explicitly communicated learning objectives guiding the debriefing. The participants' experiences of the simulation were re-actualized spontaneously. When the participants raised issues of importance for them, they constructed their own narratives, bringing back their personal experiences from the simulation as topics for reflection. The absence of structured turn-taking acted on the practice in the sense that some student sayings became foregrounded and voiced, while others were back-grounded or even silenced.

A finding coming through in students' as well as health professionals' debriefing, was the ways the material set-ups of the rooms also prefigured the unfolding of the two patterns of debriefing practice described. The set-up of the room (such as fixed positioning of chairs, tables, and participants, as well as the use of video clips demonstrating successful examples of performances of the participants) prefigured the pattern of the algorithm to be followed. Like the algorithm, the *laissez-faire* pattern of debriefing was also related to a distinct set-up of the debriefing room. In this case, the room was laid out with swivel chairs around four small round tables and a video screen on one side of the room, the video equipment was not used and not noticed by the participants and. Participants' and facilitators' positionings around the small tables were arbitrary. The material set-up of the room thereby prefigured a loosely structured and collegial debriefing practice, comprising an open invitation to participate in the reflection according to whatever the participants would like to bring up for discussion. The topics raised in the discussion by the participants, whether they were positive or negative, were emphasized by the facilitators as being valuable experiences, empowering their participation in future professional practice. Interestingly, both patterns of debriefing practice seldom explicitly thematized interprofessional collaboration and learning as a topic for reflection in the discussion even though that was one of the overall aims of the simulation activity.

7.2.6   Professionals' Debriefings: Same and Different

From our studies (Nyström et al. 2017) with professionals in interprofessional simulation-based education, we can identify some similarities with the findings from our studies of students debriefing. The focus on individual doings in relation and response to other participants and the sequence of events in the simulation was shown to be the characteristic and most common way of reflecting upon what happened in the simulation also in our study of professionals debriefing of simulation activities (Nyström et al. 2017). Like the debriefing with students, participants were instructed to think about and describe individual things they did well and individual things they could improve, based on what happened during the simulation. The instructions can be interpreted as the rules (Schatzki 2002) that compose and influence the practice of debriefing, directing the participants to perform certain actions and bring up certain topics for discussion.

The second issue that emerged as a focus for the professionals' reflections in the debriefing that resembles what we saw emerging in the students' debriefing sessions concerned the patient/manikin. Here, the sayings emphasised the medical condition, and biomedical knowledge, how it could be treated and what would constitute the correct intervention in the specific case of a patient with acute and deteriorating conditions. Reflecting upon the medical status of the patient and the appropriate treatment and behaviour can be seen as teleoaffective structures at play (Schatzki 2002) in the debriefing practice. A normative dimension of praising or correcting certain professional behaviour and performances as well as medical procedures guided the interactions at this stage. The findings of these studies support previous research (Dieckmann et al. 2009, Dismukes et al. 2006, Husebø et al. 2013) in that the facilitation of the group process plays an important role for how the debriefing emerges.

7.2.7   Debriefing with Professionals: Team-Directed Analysis

In cases where the team performance *did* emerge as a topic for discussion the descriptive focus on individual actions happening in the sequence of events in the simulation was shifted towards a team-directed analysis.

This shift was particularly noticeable emerging in the group of professionals. When a team-directed analysis emerged, the facilitator and the participants reflected upon the individual performance against the backdrop of the performance of the team, taking into account the social and material arrangements of the simulation. Three themes concerning, *communication, taking action* and *bodily positioning* then became the main focus for the reflection. When team performance was emphasised over the individual actions, knowings and leadership emerged as relational and embodied. The team enacted communication when the individual sayings (or absence of sayings) was responded to by the others in the team. These findings highlight communication as an important practice dimension of interprofessional collaboration, which has also been emphasized elsewhere (e.g. Rogers et al. 2017). Team performance was also enacted as a responsibility for taking action. These actions could be e.g. questioning or standing up for a decision, noticing when a profession's specific skills and knowledge are needed, and adopting leadership.

Last, the team also emerged as a topic for reflection through the professionals' debriefing on how bodily positionings and movements of the professional team members were enacted as a fluid chain of actions of collaboration. Interprofessional collaboration thus emerges as *more* than verbal communication. The focus on embodied professional knowings shifts the attunements from the individual doings and sayings and from primarily addressing medical aspects. Instead, interprofessional bodily actions and understandings, such as whose hands were working with what and how to anticipate the team's actions were emphasised. The activities of the chain of actions in the scenario comprised different activities, such as noticing signs indicating a deterioration of the patient's condition (auditory or visual). The noticing was followed by enactment of leadership through taking action or responding through attuning to the action of others. In the debriefing with the professionals, the facilitator directed the attunement to the priorities made by the team and probed for reflections concerning the anticipation of the next action. These probes also involved how the material arrangements were related to, and how responsibilities for different actions were distributed in the team.

7.2.8 Discussion

What are the insights for learning to be drawn from the analysis of the different debriefing practices in this subsection? Following the practice theory perspective, practices and material arrangements are relational in the sense that practices effect, give meaning to and are inseparable from material arrangements (Schatzki 2012). At the same time, material arrangements prefigure certain activities more likely to happen. Activity is not, however fixed or laid down in advance. It is only in the performance that activity becomes definite. Returning to the practice theory idea that activities of a practice is organized by rules, teleoaffective structures, practical and general understandings, we can note that the findings of our studies indicate that different sociomaterial arrangements and different practical understandings of debriefing influence participants' learning in different ways. Our findings show that a practical understanding of debriefing as *algorithm* prefigured a step-by-step sequence of the reconstruction of the sayings and doings in the scenario. The use of exemplary videoclips enabled attunement to values regarding good professional procedures and what could be taken forward to improve behaviors in a future scenario. Enacting the rules of debriefing as a step-by-step sequence, also meant that participants' own spontaneous reflections on what happened were backgrounded and less likely to emerge as a path for re-constructing the scenario.

Debriefing as *laissez-faire* on the other hand, was emerging from a different practical understanding, that prefigured participants' narratives emerging as spontaneous. The informal and open format of the debriefing session enabled the reconstruction the sequence of events in the simulation, where the structure was based on the what emerged as relevant to students' experiences in the scenario. In that sense, debriefing as *laissez-faire* seemed in our study to accommodate for reflection over individual learning needs, something that has been emphasized as important in previous research on feedback in debriefing (Motola et al. 2013). Our findings that facilitation of debriefing in a way that explicitly highlights interprofessional collaboration and learning is an issue for further research and development to improve simulation pedagogy.

The importance of reflection for learning has been, and still is, emphasized in pedagogies for professional learning, following Schön's ideas (2003). "Pedagogies of reflection" have, however, also been critiqued (Guile 2011) for being more directed towards the individual than towards the practice, and for assuming that "theoretical and practical reasoning are separate and different from one another and are best related through some reflective process" (p. 133). Guile suggests that this idea instead separates the two kinds of reasoning and maintains the idea of theoretical concepts are learned in an educational context and a 'disciplinary space of reasoning'. Another aspect of critique of the reflective paradigm that Guile puts forward, is that "professional practice is individual and profession-specific" (p. 133). He argues that in the practice field, situated judgements and decisions are carried out from a 'profession-based space of reason', and that this is what learners need to be challenged to reflect on. In an interprofessional practice, the profession-based space of reasons needs to challenge the team to reflect on how a shared space of reason was reached, where the different team members could contribute to and also evaluate the actions of others.

7.2.8.1   Implications for Practice: Situating Debriefing Into the Interprofessional Space

The findings presented in this chapter raise questions if simulation-based training serves the same purposes for students as for professionals. When comes to simulation-based education in undergraduate health care programs, it is reasonable to assume that the learners in this context differ from professional practitioners, who participate in simulation as part of their continuing education in the workplace. The health professionals are there to practice skills that they have already developed in their previous training. To the health professionals, the acute situation is familiar, but occurs less often, and hence needs to be practiced and refreshed under safe conditions. The students, on the other hand are there to develop professional skills that they have not yet fully acquired, in a practice situation that might be new to them. When we revisit the findings from studying debriefing with students and with professionals, we can notice that there are some similarities, but also some important differences. The topics emerging in the debriefing with students concerned to a large extent the biomedical knowledge and the correctness in professional behavior associated with the sequence of events unfolding in the scenario. These topics also surface in the professionals debriefing sessions as the most common. There is also a similarity in the sense that the individual actions in the scenario risk to overshadow the objective of interprofessional collaboration, that is more seldom thematized in the debriefing in both the student groups and the groups of health professionals. The debriefings with students are to a greater extent descriptive than the debriefing with the professionals. This is particularly noticeable in comparison with how the team performance is discussed by the professionals. The bundling between practice and material arrangements, and the sequence and flow of chains of actions displayed in the debriefing of health professionals team performance can potentially be valuable for the guiding of feedback on team performance also in student debriefings.

Drawing on Guile (2011), we suggest that the way of introducing the reflection should be modelled through a process of re-structuring and recontextualization. This means, that in order to improve practice, facilitation of reflection should not only include individual questions of 'what went well', 'what could have been done differently', and 'what do you bring to the next simulation exercise' but also explicitly assure that questions should assist the participants to understand and appreciate the reasons for the actions of other members of the team. Guile suggests that doing so means a re-structuring of the situation that provides an impetus for the team-members to co-mingle their perspectives (Guile 2011). The situation thereby is restructured to a relational, interprofessional space of reasoning. Rooney et al. (2015) suggest that also the material set-up should be included. The enlarged interprofessional space of reasoning provides a possibility for the team to use the restructuring to infer what might follow from the shared understanding, and re-contextualize this knowing into practice (Guile 2011). Noticing the varying forms and topics for debriefing as they unfold provides an opportunity for educators also to assess their effects. Doing so will impact on how debriefing is enacted and can also give input to how scenario designs might need to be revised, or what kinds of preparations participants need before simulation exercise (Dahlgren et al. 2016).

7.2.9 Conclusions

- Debriefing practices with students as well as with professionals unfold closely intertwined with the socio-material arrangements, the practical understandings, rules and general understandings of simulation.
- Different practical understandings prefigure the debriefing process as a step-by-step *algorithm* or as a *laissez-faire* process without a formal structure.
- Both debriefing practices with students focused primarily on biomedical knowledge and more seldomly thematised interprofessional collaboration as an explicit focus for reflection.
- Debriefing practices with professionals included themes concerning *communication, taking action* and *bodily positioning* as the main focus for the reflection.
- A renewal of the debriefing process is suggested to facilitate a shared, interprofessional perspective of the problem over individual capacities, and a re-contextualization of this perspective into interprofessional practice.

References

Alinier, G., Harwood, C., Harwood P., Montague, S., Huish, E., Ruparelia, K., Antuofermo, M. (2014). Featured article: Immersive clinical simulation in undergraduate health care interprofessional education: Knowledge and perceptions. *Clinical Simulation in Nursing*, *10*, e205–e216.

Berragan, L. (2011). Simulation: An effective pedagogical approach for nursing? *Nurse Education Today*, 31(7), 660–663.

Cheng, A., Eppich, W., Grant, V., Sherbino, J., Zendejas, B., Cook D.A. (2014). Debriefing for technology-enhanced simulation: A systematic review and meta-analysis. *Medical Education*, *48*(7), 657–66. https://doi.org/10.1111/medu.12432.

Cook, D. A., Hatala, R., Brydges, R., Zendejas, B., Szostek, J. H., Wang, A. T., … Hamstra, S. J. (2011). Technology-enhanced simulation for health professions education: A systematic review and metaanalysis. *Journal of the American Medical Association, 306*(9), 978.

Crookall, D. (2014). Engaging (in) gameplay and (in) debriefing. *Simulation & Gaming,* 45(4–5), 416–427.

Dahlgren, M. A., Fenwick, T., Hopwood, N. (2016). Theorising simulation in higher education: Difficulty for learners as an emergent phenomenon. *Teaching in Higher Education*, *21*(6), 613–627. https://doi.org/10.1080/13562517.2016.118 3620.

Dieckmann, P. (2009). Simulation settings for learning in acute medical care. In P. Dieckmann (Ed.), *Using simulations for education, training and research* (pp. 40–138). Lengerich: Pabst Science Publishers.

Dieckmann, P., Molin Friis, S., Lippert, A., Ostergaard, D. (2009). The art and science of debriefing in simulation: Ideal and practice. *Medical Teacher*, *31*(7), 287–94.

Dieckmann, P., Friis, S. M., Lippert, A., Ostergaard, D. (2012). Goals, success factors, and barriers for simulation-based learning: A qualitative interview study in health care. *Simulation & Gaming*, 43(5), 627–647.

Dismukes, R.K., Gaba, D.M., Howard, S.K. (2006). So many roads: Facilitated debriefing in healthcare. *Simulation in Healthcare: Journal of the Society for Simulation in Healthcare,* 1(1), 23–25.

Dreifuerst, K.T., Decker, S. (2012). Debriefing: An essential component for learning in simulation pedagogy. In P. R. Jeffries (Ed.), *Simulation in nursing education* (pp. 105–131). New York: National league of nursing.

Fanning, R.M., Gaba, D.M. (2007). The Role of debriefing in simulation-based learning. *Simulation in Healthcare,* (2), 115–25.

Gardner, R. (2013). Introduction to debriefing. *Seminars in Perinatology*, 37, 166–174.

Gough, S., Hellaby, M., Jones, N., MacKinnon, R. (2012). A review of undergraduate interprofessional simulation-based education (IPSE*). Collegian,* 19, 153–170.

Guile, D. (2011). Interprofessional activity in the "space of reasons": Thinking, communicating and acting. *Vocations and Learning,* 4(2), 93–111.

Husebø, S., Dieckmann, P., Rystedt, H., Friberg, F. (2013). The relationship between facilitators' questions and the level of reflection in the post-simulation debriefing. *Simulation in Healthcare,* 8(3), 135–142.

Jeffries, P. (2013) *Clinical Simulations in Nursing Education: Advanced Concepts, Trends, and Opportunities.* New York: National league of nursing.

Kihlgren, P., Spanager, L., Dieckmann, P. (2015). Investigating novice doctors' reflections in debriefings after simulation scenarios. *Medical Teacher, 37*(5), 437–43. https://doi.org/10.3109/0142159X.2014.956054.

Motola, I., Devine, L.A., Chung, H.S., Sullivan, J.E., Issenberg, S.B. (2013). Simulation in healthcare education: A best evidence practical guide. *Medical Teacher, 35*(10), 1511–30. https://doi.org/10.3109/0142159X.2013.818632.

Neill, M.A., Wotton, K. (2011). High-fidelity simulation debriefing in nursing education: A literature review. *Clinical Simulation in Nursing,* 7(5), e161–e168.

Nyström, S., Dahlberg J., Hult, H., Abrandt Dahlgren, M. (2016a). Observing of interprofessional collaboration in simulation: A socio-material approach. *Journal of Interprofessional Care,* 30(6), 710–716.

Nyström, S., Dahlberg, J., Edelbring, S., Hult, H., Dahlgren, M.A. (2016b). Debriefing practices in interprofessional simulation with students: A sociomaterial perspective. *BMC Medical Education,* 16, 148. https://doi.org/10.1186/s12909-016-0666-5.

Nyström S., Dahlberg J., Edelbring S., Hult H., Abrandt Dahlgren M. (2017). Continuing professional development: Pedagogical practices of interprofessional simulation in health care. *Studies in Continuing Education,* 39(3), 303–319.

Palaganas, J.C., Epps, C., Reamer, D. (2014). A history of simulation-enhanced interprofessional education. *Journal of Interprofessional Care,* 28(2), 110–115.

Poikela, P., Teräs, M. (2015). A scoping review: Conceptualizations and pedagogical models of learning in nursing simulation. *Educational Research and Reviews,* 10(8), 1023–1033.

Raemer, D., Anderson, M., Cheng, A., Ganning, R., Nadkarni, V., Salvodelli, G. (2011). Research regarding debriefing as part of the learning process. *Simulation in Healthcare,* 6(7), 52–57.

Rogers, G.D., Thistlethwaite, J.E., Anderson, E.S., Abrandt Dahlgren, M., Grymonpre, R. E., Moran, M., Samarasekera, D.D. (2017). International consensus statement on the assessment of interprofessional learning outcomes, Medical Teacher, *39*(4), 347–359. https://doi.org/10.1080/0142159X.2017.1270441.

Rooney, D., Hopwood, N., Boud, D., Kelly, M. (2015). The role of simulation in pedagogies of higher education for the health professions: Through a practice-based lens. *Vocations and Learning,* 8(3), 269–285.

Rudolph, J.W., Simon, R., Dufresne, R.L., Raemer, D.B. (2006). There's no such thing as "nonjudgmental" debriefing: A theory and method for debriefing with good judgment. *Simulation in Healthcare,* 1(1), 49–55.

Rudolph, J. W., Simon, R., Raemer, D. B., Eppich, W. J. (2008). Debriefing as formative assessment: Closing performance gaps in medical education. *Academic Emergency Medicine, 15*(11), 1010–1016. https://doi.org/10.1111/j.1553-2712.2008.00248.x.

Schatzki, T. (2002). *The site of the social: A philosophical account of the constitu-tion of social life and change.* University Park: Pennsylvania State University Press.

Schatzki, T.R. (2012). A primer on practices. In J. Higgs, R. Barnett, S. Billett, M. Hutchings & F. Trede. (Eds.), *Practice-Based Education: Perspectives and Strategies* (pp. 13–26). Rotterdam: Sense Publishers.

Sawyer, T., Eppich, W., Brett-Fleegler, M., Grant, V., Cheng, A. (2016). More than one way to debrief a critical review of healthcare simulation debriefing methods. *Journal of the Society for Simulation in Healthcare,* 11(3), 209–217.

Singh, H., Kalani, M., Acosta-Torres, S., El Ahmadieh, T.Y., Loya, J., Ganju, A. (2013). History of simulation in medicine: From Resusci Annie to the Ann Myers Medical Center. *Neurosurgery,* 73(4), 9–14.

Schön, D. A. (2003). The reflective practitioner: How professionals think in action. Aldershot: Arena.

Steinwachs, B. (1992). How to facilitate a debriefing. *Simulation & Gaming,* 23(2), 186–195.

7.3   Video as a Tool for Feedback and Reflection in Interprofessional Simulation

Elin Nordenström · Torben Nordahl Amorøe · Hans Rystedt
University of Gothenburg
Gothenburg, Sweden
e-mail: elin.nordenstrom@ped.gu.se; torben.nordahl-amoroe@vgregion.se;
hans.rystedt@ped.gu.se

7.3.1   Introduction

In this section we will present and discuss how video can be used as a tool for feed-back and reflection in post-scenario debriefing to support interprofessional learning. Video is used for feedback purposes in many educational settings, for instance sports, teacher training, medical training and simulator training. An argument for using video performance review in post-scenario debriefings is to promote collab-orative learning (Eppich et al. 2015). Video is thought to allow for a distanced and objective view of "what really happened", encourage self-reflection, help to gain insights on one's own actions – what needs to be improved or modified. Or as Fanning and Gaba, (2007, p. 122) put it:

> Video playback may be useful for adding perspective to a simulation, to allow participants to see how they performed rather than how they thought they performed, and to help reduce hindsight bias in assessment of the scenario.

Largely, the benefits of using video in simulation debriefings, as well as in other educational settings, seems to be taken for granted. This despite to the fact that there are a few empirical studies demonstrating the efficacy of video as a tool for feedback and reflection on an individual or team level. Whilst some studies have concluded that video-assisted debriefing have the potential to enhance individual skills and communication (e.g. de Vita et al. 2005; Grant et al. 2010; Hamilton et al. 2011), others have failed to demonstrate any significant effects of video-assisted debriefing compared to other forms of debriefing (e.g. Savoldelli et al. 2006). Some have also pointed out that the difficulties in finding univocal effects depend on the problems to assess and compare outcomes between a rather wide range of interventions (Ali and Miller 2018). Following the theoretical approach in video studies of situated actions (see Chap. 2, this volume), we argue that answering the question of whether video is effective or not need requires additional empirical studies that are sensitive to the complexity and details involved in its practical use in everyday debriefing practices.

Based on guidelines in handbooks and best practice manuals for educational practitioners, there seems to be a general understanding of video recordings as capturing "everything as it is", and thus constituting complete and objective representations of the recorded educational activities. With this follows the assumption that video recordings are "self-explaining". That is, learners watching the recordings can easily understand what they are meant to show and discern relevant aspects of educational or professional conduct. This view is, however, challenged by a number of studies demonstrating that video in itself is not sufficient to enhance the understanding and contribute to insights on one's own or others' professional conduct. In a study of video use in teacher training Erickson (2007) shows that the students when asked to observe and comment on a video recording of a teaching episode largely came up with superficial observations of aspects that were not professionally relevant. As maintained by Erickson, novices watching video without guidance tend to "find themselves at sea, in a stream of continuous detail they don't know how to parse during the course of their real-time viewing in order to make sense of it" (p. 146). A conclusion drawn from the study is that instructional guidance is of vital importance to direct the learners' attention towards relevant details of the recording and unpack how these are meant to be understood. Similar findings are presented by studies in the field of dental education, showing how the students' possibilities to make sense of root canal treatments displayed on video are highly dependent on the comments and questions from instructors and their use of video to constitute a shared point of reference (Lindwall et al. 2014; Lindwall and Lymer 2014; Rystedt et al. 2013). A classical study by Goodwin (1994) on video as evidence in courtrooms, provides a good example of the extent to which expert guidance can be crucial for how observers understand the course of events in a video recording. The study demonstrates how expert witnesses' instructions through talk and gestures shaped the ways in which jury members interpreted video recordings of policemen's use of violence against a suspect. By highlighting specific occurrences in the video and explain in detail how these were to be interpreted from a professional point of view, the experts were able to convince jury members to understand a rather obvious instance of police brutality as a case of appropriate professional work (the case was later subject to another trial in which this standpoint was rejected). Similar findings have been reached by studies of video use in other domains. A study of reality TV parenting shows (McIlvenny 2011), for instance, shows how professionals use video recordings to confront parents with evidence of their own unsuccessful behavior towards their children. Also, in this case, selection of episodes, highlighting of specific occurrences, and instructions by the professionals greatly influences how the video recordings are understood by those who observe them. In sum, these studies show how a certain understanding of video recordings can be provided through talk and gestures, and how the additional perspective provided by the video can be consequential for subsequent activities.

Against this backdrop, we have developed empirically grounded guidelines for how video can be used as a tool for feedback and reflection in interprofessional simulation. Firstly, we have developed a model for how video sequences can be introduced by facilitators *prior* to the displaying to create favorable conditions for student reflection, and secondly, we show how facilitators' questions *after* the displaying can guide the students' understanding of interprofessional teamwork, as shown on video recorded scenarios.

7.3.2 The Empirical Case and Methods

The chapter is based on two data sets: (1) data from a collaborative video workshop with the research group and facilitators from the simulation center, and (2) video recordings of 8 1-day interprofessional simulation training occasions including a total of 40 simulation sessions for nursing and medical students in the final phases of their educational programs. The video workshop formed the basis for the development of guidelines on how to introduce video clips, and the video recordings were used as basis for the guidelines on how to promote reflection after the viewing of video clips.

The goal of the recorded simulation training was to increase the competencies needed for efficient management of emergency situations in multi-professional teams. Four main goals were defined out of the CRM (Crisis Resource Management) and ATLS (Advanced Trauma Life Support) principles. These were structured examination in line with the *ABCDE-sequence* (Airway, Breathing, Circulation, Disability, Environment); reporting and communication of patient status in accordance with the *SBAR* reporting system (Situation, Background, Assessment, Recommendation); *Closed loops* to ensure effective communication with feedback; and *Speak up* to emphasize the responsibility of all team members to communicate important information such as concerns, warnings and suggestions.

The simulations were designed in line with the guidelines for simulation training in healthcare as suggested by Dieckmann et al. (2017) and others, implying a three-phase model: *briefing, scenario* and *debriefing*. A 1-hour lecture preceded the simulation training, emphasizing principles for teamwork, structured communication and systematic management of patients in potentially life-threatening situations.

The briefings consisted of short introductions to the scenarios, which comprised common medical conditions in various healthcare settings that the students were likely to meet in their professional career. The debriefing followed the widespread model originally developed by Steinwachs (1992) implying a three-step procedure: description, analysis and application. Firstly, when the trainees gathered after the scenario, they were asked to express their immediate feeling (blow out) and then to provide a brief and factual description of what happened (description phase). This was followed by a second step, involving a discussion of what went well during the scenario and what could be improved (analysis phase). The third step aimed at drawing conclusions on what could be learnt from the exercise (application phase).

Briefings, scenarios and debriefings were recorded with one to two video cameras (see Chap. 3a for a description of the recording process) and the recordings were partially transcribed according to the conventions developed by Jefferson (1984). In Table 7.1, explanations of the transcript conventions used in this chapter are presented.

The recordings were subject to close interaction analysis informed by ethnomethodology and conversation analysis (Heath et al. 2010; see Chap. 2, this volume).

The joint video workshop was arranged in line with guidelines for video data sessions within the social sciences (Derry et al. 2010; Heath et al. 2010). As maintained by Heath et al. (2010) practitioners, that is, personnel from the research domain, can often make valuable contributions in data sessions by providing "distinct insights... and... help to clarify events that have proved difficult to understand" (p. 102). The three facilitators participating in the workshop had extensive experience of leading debriefings, and they had all experience of using video as a means for feedback and reflection. Moreover, as senior physicians and nurses they could contribute with valuable domain-related expertise that the researchers did not have. A recommendation by Heath et al. (ibid.) is to avoid overwhelming participants in data sessions with too much materials, but instead concentrate on a small number of brief extracts. For the present workshop, one of the researchers (EN) selected three extracts that were subject to detailed and collaborative scrutiny. The discussion was recorded and after the workshop the researchers summarized the analytical observations. These observations formed the basis for further analytical work by the researchers.

Table 7.1 Transcript conventions used in this chapter

[word]	Syllables or word/s within brackets are overlapping with another speaker's talk (also within brackets)
=	Shows that two utterances are latched, i.e. there is no pause between the utterances
(.)	Micropause, shorter than 0.2 s
(1.4)	Length in absolute seconds of gap or pause longer than 0.2 s between words or turns
Word	Underlining indicates emphasis (here of the first two syllables of the word)
WORD	Word/s in capitals is pronounced louder than surrounding speech by the same speaker
Word-	Talk is cut-off
(word)	Indicates that the transcriber is uncertain of the word. Empty brackets or xxx within the brackets represents inaudible speech
((word))	Text within double brackets is transcriber's description of gaze or bodily actions conducted meanwhile the utterance on the line above is produced

7.3.3 Using Open-Ended or Specific Introductions to Video?

As suggested in literature on simulation-based health care education, video-feedback as a component of debriefings facilitates and guides reflection (e.g. Dieckmann et al. 2008; Eppich et al. 2015, Fanning and Gaba 2007). This, however, with the reservation that there is a lack of hands-on recommendations on how to integrate video in debriefings. Addressing this need, the research group in collaboration with experienced debriefing facilitators in a first step developed practical guidelines for how to select video-clips from recordings of simulation scenarios to be displayed to learners in debriefing, and how to relate the viewing of these clips to the prevailing debriefing model. The work by the research group and the facilitators were informed by principles for collaborative analyses of video data (see Heath et al. 2010), and by prior experiences of integrating video in debriefings at the simulator center. A first step was to determine criteria for selection of video clips and decide on in what stage of the debriefings the clips would be shown. The researchers and the facilitators jointly concluded that the four goals of the simulation training listed above should be used as basis for selection. Moreover, the clips should be brief enough to enable focused discussions (<1 min). The clips should be introduced as a first step of the second phase (analysis) in the debriefing model, that is, when addressing what had worked well in the scenario. This implied that the clips should exemplify well-functioning aspects of teamwork, which in turn, were intended to provide a basis for furthering discussions on what could be improved and learnt.[1]

In a next stage, the research group and three of the most experienced facilitators at the center arranged a joint video workshop (see Heath et al. 2010) to develop a model for how to introduce selected video clips to learners to promote reflection. From a review of the 40 recorded debriefings, each between 30 and 40 min in length, 3 examples of introductions of video clips were selected by one of the researchers (EN). Based on the researcher's analysis of the recorded debriefings, the examples were intended to illustrate three types of introductions: highly structured, mid-structured and less structured.

During the video workshop, the three examples of introductions were displayed to the facilitators who were asked to grade them individually on a 10-grade scale with the end-points "open-ended" (1) and "specific" (10). All three facilitators graded the introductions in similar ways, which largely matched the grading done by the researcher. In the introduction regarded as most *open-ended* the students were told to attend to "an instance of good communication". Whilst this introduction gave a hint on what to attend to when watching the clip, communication is a rather open notion which meant that it was largely left to the students to discern what aspects of the video clip were relevant to focus and reflect upon. In contrast, the introduction regarded as most *specific* was characterized by detailed information about the situation displayed in the video clip and instructions on what details of the

---

[1] A corresponding design has been applied at Copenhagen Academy for Medical Education and Simulation (CAMES) and by Savoldelli et al. (2006).

situation to focus and reflect upon. This introduction premised more explicitly to look for what information a team member got about the patient case when entering the ward room to assist with the ongoing examination. The introduction pointed out both a certain point of time and what was said about the patient's condition, which placed this form of introduction in the more specific end of the scale.

Very open ended and very specific introductions are at opposite ends of the scale, but there were also middle ways variations on the scale. One of the clips were assessed as middle range. In contrast to open-ended introductions, the facilitators meant that such a middle way is characterized by giving a more delineated topic. In this case as the facilitator expressed that she would like to show "a good example of structured teamwork". As concluded by the facilitators in the video workshop, "structured teamwork" is rather open-ended, but still more specific than "good communication" and less specific than the instruction to look for the information that is provided at a given point of time.

After the grading of the examples, a joint discussion took place to reach an agreement on what was the criteria for open-ended and specific introductions, respectively. During this discussion a range of various strategies for introducing video clips were identified, ranging from being rather specific to rather open-ended. The end-point "open-ended" were interpreted as giving no information at all except for showing a video-clip and "specific" to present exactly what actions to observe and the reasons for doing so. The end-points were thoroughly ruled out as appropriate alternatives but were referred to as reference points for labelling and characterizing the various ways of introducing video clips.

Next, the facilitators were shown how the debriefings unfolded after the different kinds of introductions. Based on this, the facilitators were requested to discuss the implications of open versus specific introductions for the students' discussions and reflections on the video clips. The discussion was closely related to the facilitators' views on how debriefings should be designed to approach the learning objectives. They emphasized that the selected clips should function as a *shared point of reference* for students to reflect on the *consequences* of their actions in the simulation scenarios and to connect to general *principles of teamwork*. In all, this puts demands on selecting clips on the fly that not only show something significant about teamwork, but also could show something that could promote focused discussions.

Both advantages and disadvantages with the different forms of introductions were identified. On the one hand, a specific introduction could contribute to students' confidence, but on the other, it could constrain the students' possibilities for reflections and bringing up their own concerns. As one of the facilitators put it, "I want a direction, so they have something to direct their attention to... not too specific though because I want them to discover things as well". This implied decisions on whether the reason of introducing and showing the video clip was to assure a focus on relevant aspects of teamwork or if it was intended for students to make discoveries on their own. In all, the discussion turned out in an agreement on that both forms of introductions have advantages and disadvantages, which are summarized below (Fig. 7.1).

As illustrated by Fig. 7.1, both open-ended and specific introductions have advantages and disadvantages. After the video workshop, the researcher group summarized the results of the discussions based on a recording of the workshop. This resulted in a model including a number of more context dependent principles for how to decide on when to use open-ended, semi open-ended or specific introductions, respectively, when presenting video-clips to learners. These are:

1. *Situation in the video clip* – is the situation clear for the students, unclear or somewhere in between? For instance, when showing a sequence of applying ABCDE, it is often an obvious focus for students' focus, whilst when showing an instance of communication in general, it might be rather vague for the students' what facet of the activities to attend to.
2. *Purpose* – what is expected to achieve by showing the video clip? Do you want to give the participants an aha-experience, encourage them or give an example of what works well or what can be improved?
3. *Time* – is it the first scenario in the morning, the middle of the day or is it late in the afternoon? The moment of time in the training has consequences for how familiar the participants are with each other, the facilitator and the debriefing structure, and how alert they are.
4. *Group/atmosphere* – is it for instance a talkative or a quiet group? On the one hand, if the group is rather reluctant to voice their ideas, more specific introductions could offer a clearer frame for what is expected and a certain topic to align to. On the other hand, an open-ended introduction in a talkative group could offer opportunities to a freer exploration of the students' own concerns.

The four principles presented above imply that a range of aspects have to be considered when choosing how to introduce video clips *before* they are displayed. The

	ADVANTAGE	DISADVANTAGE
OPEN	Learners get the opportunity to discover and reflect independently of the facilitator	Learners focus more on technical skills than teamwork Risk that learners focus on other (negative) aspects in the video clip than what was intended by the facilitator
SPECIFIC	Learners feel more secure Helps learners to identify relevant aspects of teamwork	Video clip provides no "aha-experience" Risk that learners only focus on aspects that the facilitator asks about

Fig. 7.1 Advantages and disadvantages of using open-ended versus specific introductions

next section will address how learners' understanding of video recorded interprofessional teamwork can be guided through the facilitators' questions and contributions from peers *after* the displaying of video clips. Whilst the principles for introducing video clips were developed through a collaborative video workshop involving researchers and facilitators, these guidelines are based on an in-depth interaction analysis of the video recordings of the debriefings undertaken by the researchers.

7.3.4 Can Video Support Discussion and Reflection?

To explore in what ways video-use could promote reflections on interprofessional teamwork the researchers undertook a close analysis of the 40 video recorded debriefings. The focus was put on episodes that took place immediately *after* a video clip had been displayed and instances in which the video was explicitly referred to in the discussion. More specifically, the analysis was guided by an interest for how the students talked about their own and other students' performance as displayed on video, and how the facilitators' questions and instructions guided the students' contributions and shaped their understandings of the displayed instances.

In the following, two episodes are presented that showcase how video clips (A) provide a visual display for taking a third-person perspective on what took place in the scenario and (B) a means for contrasting visual appearance against first-person experiences of the scenario.

Episode 1 presented in Fig. 7.2, shows a sequence from a debriefing that takes place after the students have watched a brief video clip of the recording of the scenario and are asked by one of the facilitators (FA2) leading the debriefing to identify positive aspects of teamwork. The episode illustrates how a topic is introduced by the facilitator with reference to the clip, and how this is responded to by the students.

In line 108–109 we can see how the facilitator reveals the intention of displaying the video clip, that is, to *show* how the students" work together". The following question (line 111–113) is like the preceding utterance phrased in terms of how the situation appears visually: "...did you *see* something...". In this way, the question makes relevant for an answer phrased in terms of what can be *seen* and *heard* in the video clip. Moreover, the formulation of the question presumes a focus on positive aspects of the video clip: in line with the debriefing model's focus on what went well the facilitator asks if the students see something they think works *well* (line 113).

As can be seen from the nursing student's response beginning on line 117, the question is understood as a request for a positive assessment of the team's and her own performance *as it appears on the video*. The student begins by commenting on the team's joint behaviors in positive terms: "we looked *calm*", "we were talking *loud*". Note here that talking loudly is framed as something positive, that is, a way to communicate in a clear and audible way rather than yelling in an upset manner. Calm and structured manners and clear communication are both relevant aspects of

```
108    FA2:    We want- we want to show a little about
109            how you work together
110                (0.6)
111    FA2:    what what (do you) thi- did you see
112            something that you think
113            works well here
114                (0.4)
115    NU1:    (.mph)
116                (3.0)
117    NU1:    So (0.6) I think it nevertheless looks
118            like b- eh we look sort of
119            uh (.) .ptk calm we stand around the
120            patient 'n' like talking loud but not in
121            an unpleasant way for the patient not sort
122            of like this oh my god how [but]
123    NU5:                               [nah]
124    NU1:    more like this (.) yeah but now have we
125            how has he peed now have you pee-
126            so like this 'n' (.) I saw on myself that
127            it- I nevertheless thought I looked nice
128            there when I stood 'n'
129            [LISTENED TO YOU SOMEHOW]
130    NU2:    [ah-HA-HA hahaha          ]
131    NU1:    =I looked calm I held the patient but at
132            the same time I was very like
133            attentive to (0.5) to listen to what we
134            said it felt like we were there somehow
135    NU3:    m
```

Fig. 7.2 Episode 1 – taking a third-person perspective on one's own actions

teamwork, and something that has been stressed in the lecture prior to the simulation sessions.

In line 126 the student continues to comment on her own behavior saying that she "looked nice". In contrast to her previous comment, this one is treated by the other students as something humorous and laughable (line 130), possibly because "I looked nice" can be understood as a praise of the student's personal characteristic rather than an assessment of her professional teamwork skills. As seen in line 131 the nursing student does not join in the laughter, however, but provides an account that justifies the positive self-talk. The student says that she "looked calm" and that she was "attentive" to listen to what the other students said. Unlike "I looked nice" these attributes are relevant aspects of teamwork, and also are treated as such by the other students who stop laughing and provide affirmative responses.

If we turn back to how the discussion started and look at the entire episode, we can see that the video rather than the students' recollected experiences is used as a ground for commenting on the students' performance in the displayed situation. The facilitator's question after the displaying of the video clip servers to establish a focus on *visual* and *audible* aspects of the situation: "did you *see* something that you think works well here". This focus is then maintained by the nursing student's response that highlights aspects of her own and the other students' performance that can be *seen* and *heard*. First the "we *looked* sort of calm" and "[we were] talking *loud*" in line 117–120, and then the "I *looked* calm" and "I was very like attentive" on line 131–133. What is notable here is that the video and the facilitator's instructional guidance provide a necessary resource for discerning this kind of visual and audible aspect of the own and other's performance. Looking at how oneself acts and interacts with other team members from a distanced perspective is not possible while performing the scenario, but necessitates an additional third-person view of the situation, one that is here provided by the video. The video in itself does not direct the students' attentions towards the visual and audible aspects of their behavior, however, but the facilitator's question after the displaying of the clip is crucial for this matter.

The second episode (Fig. 7.3) shows how the video serves as a resource for contrasting visual appearance against first-person experiences of the displayed situation. Like the previous episode, this one shows a discussion that takes place immediately after the displaying of a video clip. Two of the nursing students (NU2 and NU3) and one medical student (ME1) took part in the scenario while the other students followed it via live-video from the debriefing room. The discussion in episode 2 (Fig. 7.3) relates to an issue that was addressed at an earlier stage of the debriefing conversation; in the beginning of the debriefing the students were asked how they felt after the scenario. The students said that they felt insecure, insufficient and blocked, and it appeared that they regarded their performance as far too passive during the scenario.

The question asked by the facilitator after the displaying of the video clip invites for an assessment of the atmosphere in the simulation room. The answer, "it was very calm", is initially provided by a nursing student (NU1) who did not take part in the simulation scenario, but observed it via video. Her response thus provides an observer's perspective of the situation in a double sense: first, she observed the scenario as it played out in real-time, and then she observed the selected video clip in the debriefing. Another of the students, NU2, who *did* take part in the scenario and thus have both first-hand experience and an observer's perspective of the displayed situation adds that this is how it *looked* on the video at least, and then laughs: "yeah it really looked that way on the video at least" (line 208–209). A medical student (ME1) who also took part in the scenario, joins in the laughter and then says that it "looked very relaxed", referring to the situation as displayed on video. From the students' comments and laughter, it appears that they, as having dual perspectives of the situation, perceive a contrast between how the situation *appears visually* and how it was *experienced* it in real-time; *looking* calm and relaxed do not necessarily mean *being* calm and relaxed.

In lines 214–219, the facilitator joins in and first reminds the students of their reported feelings immediately after the scenario – ME1 felt insufficient, NU2 insecure, and NU3 blocked – after which she adds "'n' so we look at the clip" (line 221) thus highlighting the video as the common point of reference for further discussions. Just like the students, the facilitator thus points to the contrast between the students' *experience* of the scenario and the *appearance* of it as available to every-

```
201    FAC:    What did you think about the atmosphere in
202            the room then?
203                (2.7)
204    NU1:    It was very calm
205    FAC:    m?=
206    NU1:    =m
207                (0.7)
208    NU2:    yeah it really looked that £on the video
209            [at least    ]£
               ((said with smiley voice and embedded
                laughter))
210    ME1:    [yeah-he-he-he]
211    FAC:    yeah?
212    ME1:    £it (was) very (.) relaxed
213    NU2:    yeah=
214    FAC:    =yeah 'n' what do you think about that I
215            think then ge- we return to those
216            feelings that you had when you (.) 'n' so
217            (ME1) you thought you were insufficient
218            'n' (NU2) you said you were insecure 'n'
219            (NU3) were blocked 'n'
220                (1.8)
221            'n' so we look at the clip
222                (0.9)
223    ME1:    uh (.) (naha)
224                (1.4)
225    NU1:    it didn't show on you
226    NU2:    nah
227    NU1:    it wasn't outwardly noticeable (0.6) as a
228            patient I think one would have felt calm
229            'n' safe
230                (1.1)
231            in this
232                (0.8)
233    FAC:    yeah how do you think (0.3) when you see
234            this
235                (2.7)
236    NU2:    Yeah I don't think that feeling is (.)
237            like reflected in the clip- like one-
238            it's not outwardly visible
239    FAC:    nah?
```

Fig. 7.3 Episode 2 – reconceptualizing experiences

one via the video, however, making another point out of this; while the students made the point that the visual appearance of the situation was misleading since it did not correspond with how they experienced it, the facilitator seems to suggest that the visual appearance is what counts. After a short pause, the nursing students (NU1) who was the first to respond to the facilitator's question about the atmosphere, responds by elaborating on the perspective introduced by the facilitator: "it didn't show on you" (line 225), and then, "it wasn't outwardly noticeable (0.6) as a patient I think one would have felt calm 'n' safe" (line 227–229). The point made by the facilitator and the observing student here is that the students' reported experiences were not visible – neither to them as observers nor the patient – but as it appeared from the video clip the atmosphere was calm and the students attended to the patient in a professional way. Turning towards the students who took part in the scenario the facilitator goes on to ask: "yeah how do you think when you see this?". The question is responded by the nursing students (NU2) who earlier pointed to the contrast between how the situation appeared and how she had experienced it. The answer is in line with the perspective introduced by the facilitator, "Yeah I don't think that feeling is like reflected in the clip- like one- it's not outwardly visible" (line 236–238), which suggests that the student, if not having re-evaluated the situation, is now at least is able to see it from the perspective introduced by the facilitator. To this, the facilitator provides a strong confirmative response and moves on to a next question which suggests that she is satisfied with the outcome of the discussion.

In summary, Episode 2 (Fig. 7.3) shows how the students' understanding of the video clip is re-conceptualized in three step process. Firstly, the facilitator emphasizes the contrast between the students' reported feelings and the visual in the video clip. Secondly the facilitators' point is elaborated by one of the observing students, and thirdly, this point of view is acknowledged by one of the students who took part in the scenario.

7.3.5   Discussion

This chapter has described the development of practical guidelines for introducing video clips and explored possibilities and challenges involved in following up of video clips displayed in post-scenario debriefings with the intention to promote discussion and reflection on interprofessional teamwork. This work was done in two steps: through a collaborate video workshop with researchers and facilitators, and through interaction analysis of video recorded debriefings.

A major outcome from the video workshop was a conceptual model aimed to support debriefing facilitators' selection and framing of video clips that is sensitive to the context at hand: i.e. the situation, purpose, point of time and group/atmosphere. Further, the workshop served to highlight the importance of selecting clips that could serve as a context for discussing the consequences of the team members' joint actions and behaviors on a detailed level. In this way, the idea was that more general aspects of importance for interprofessional teamwork could be addressed. This assumption is to a large extent confirmed through the detailed interaction analysis of the video recordings of the debriefings. Although interprofessional learning, that is, learning from and with each other, was the goal of the training, it was not brought up as a concept *per se*. However, the analysis of the 40 video-recorded debriefings shows that facilitators and students recurrently raised issues that fall under CRM and ATLS guidelines, such as maintaining a shared view of the situation and coordinating the workflow in a structured manner. In the episodes provided here, topics as being attentive to other team-members actions (Episode 1) and working in a calm and systematic manner (Episode 2), exemplifies how central aspects of teamwork are made relevant through the interplay between the facilitators' questions and the student responses.

The conclusions in the workshop on when to use open-ended versus specific introductions can be further nuanced by looking at conversation analytic research on feedback and assessment in the area of higher and professional education. Whilst there is a well-established expectation that open-ended questions give students the freedom to address concerns and problems in their own terms, empirical studies have shown open questions to produce unelaborated responses that do not further the dialogue (e.g. Hofvendahl 2006). When it comes to open questions requesting assessment of the own performance, these have shown to be even more ineffective. Waring (2014) shows that students when invited in open terms to assess their own performances appeared to understand the questions as a form of test and withheld their responses to avoid the risk of coming up with assessments that did not match the teachers' agenda. In short, this research strengthens the conclusions from the workshop that open-ended questions might not always promote reflection and that more specific introductions would be preferable if the group feels reluctant or if it is unclear for the students what facets of the shown situation to attend to.

The interaction analysis of how discussions developed after the displaying of video clips illustrates that video is a powerful tool that can encourage discussions and reflections in various ways. Most important, the video enables for observations from *a third-person perspective*. Without the video it would not have been possible for the students to observe the actual appearance of their own conduct. Neither would it have been possible to assess the communication and interaction with the other students in the scenario. Although it is not obvious in the examples presented here, students regularly report that they do not remember what they actually did during the scenario and that they had another perspective of time, something that the video-clips gave them a more realistic perception of (see Oxelmark et al. 2017).

Watching video has an instructional function during debriefings. The video is used as instructional means in the sense that students are encouraged to look for what worked well, but also to re-evaluate their performance in terms of its visible consequences for teamwork (see McIlvenny 2011). The students are guided to focus on how things look and sound in the video, and the looks are tied to professional conduct, both by the students and the facilitators. It can also be seen, especially in the second example, that the video can function as visual evidence that take precedence over the reported experiences/feelings. In the current example, this can be regarded as highly relevant for interprofessional teamwork. With the help of the video the facilitator could give another perspective of the situation and show that the students' strongly self-critical attitude, which was a recurrent theme in all 40 video recorded debriefings, was actually ungrounded – even though they felt that they have performed poorly the video showed that they handled the situation in a professional way. When using video, however, it is important to highlight both the experienced and visual perspective of the situation, that is, not assigning the video with the status of the "true burden of proof". How a clinical situation appears from a third-person perspective is important indeed – that is the perspective of patients, dependents, and co-workers – but so are experiences of the medical practitioners. An assurance that one was able to maintain a professional face despite inner feelings of stress, insecurity and insufficiency might not be enough to boost self-esteem, but there might be a need to also address why such feelings have emerged and how they should be handled.

Interprofessional learning takes on two quite distinct meanings here (Johansson et al. 2017). On the one hand, the debriefings are designed to learn from each other about interprofessional teamwork through the joint analysis of the events shown in the recordings. On the other hand, how to collaborate in professional teams is what the students should learn from the scenarios, and is of central concern in the students and facilitators discussions.

To summarize, the video is central as a basis for discussion and reflections, but it does not itself guarantee that inexperienced participants discern interprofessionally relevant aspects by themselves. Instead, the instructors' guidance is critical for the students to see the recorded events in a particular way that is relevant for coordinated teamwork; or, as Goodwin (1994) points out in his study of professional vision, how experts organize "the perceptual field provided by the videotape into a salient figure" (p. 620). But the power of video to shape the students' understanding of interprofessional teamwork also put extensive demands on facilitators to select appropriate clips on the fly in the midst of ongoing scenarios. It could be especially challenging to, simultaneously, identify situations that illustrate important facets of interprofessional teamwork, which, in addition could work as candidates for encouraging discussions and reflections. For these reasons, the optimal use of video might be a rather challenging task for facilitators, demanding a great deal of experience. But we also think it is something that could benefit from collaborative reviewing and reflections on the facilitators own debriefings in the ways presented in this chapter.

7.3.6 Conclusions

- The use of open-ended versus specific introduction to video-clips in debriefings should take into consideration the situation to be shown, the purpose, the point of time and the group/atmosphere.
- The use of video in debriefings enables the re-actualization of prior events and could provide a third-person perspective on the teams' own conduct
- Video can function as a means for re-conceptualizing how the participants' conduct is to be seen and assessed in relation to the demands of interprofessional teamwork
- The instructors' guidance is decisive for students' possibilities to see and understand the recorded events in ways that are relevant for professional conduct

- The results underline that the successful use of video relies on to what extent the instructional design and methods in use are sensitive to the concrete conditions for students to understand and develop interprofessional competencies

References

Ali, A.A., Miller, E.T. (2018). Effectiveness of video-assisted debriefing in health education: An integrative review. *Journal of Nursing Education*, 57(1), 14–20.

Dieckmann, P., Reddersen, S., Zieger, J., & Rall, M. (2008). A structure for video-assisted debriefing in simulator-based training of crisis resource management. In R. Kyle & B. W. Murray (Eds.), *Clinical Simulation: Operations, Engineering, and Management* (pp. 667–676). Burlington: Academic.

Dieckmann, P., Molin Friis, S., Lippert, A., Østergaard, D. (2017). Goals, success factors, and barriers for simulation-based learning: A qualitative interview study in health care. *Simulation & Gaming,* 43(5), 627–647.

Eppich, W.J., Hunt, E.A., Duval-Arnould, J.M., Sidall, V.J., Cheng, A. (2015). Structuring feedback and debriefing to achieve mastery learning goals. *Academic Medicine*, 90(11), 1501–1511.

Erickson, F. (2007). Ways of seeing video: Towards a phenomenology of viewing minimally edited footage. In R. Goldman, R. Pea, S. Barron & S. Derry (Eds.), *Video research in the learning sciences* (pp. 145–155). Mahwah: Lawrence Erlbaum Associate Publishers.

De Vita, M.A., Schaefer, J.L., Wang, H., Dongilli, T. (2005). Improving emergency medical (MED) team performance using a novel curriculum and a computerized human patient simulator. *Quality and Safety Health Care*, 14, 326–331.

Derry, S.J., Pea, R.D., Barron, B., Engle, R.A., Erickson, F., Goldman, R., et al. (2010). Conducting video research in the learning sciences: Guidance on selection, analysis, technology, and ethics. *The Journal of the Learning Sciences*, 19(1), 3–53.

Fanning, R.M., Gaba, D.M. (2007). The role of debriefing in simulation-based learning. *Simulation in Healthcare*, 2(2), 115–125.

Goodwin, C. (1994). Professional vision. *American Anthropologist, 96*(3), 606–633.

Grant, J.S., Moss, J., Epps, C., Watts, P. (2010). Using video-facilitated feedback to improve student performance following high-fidelity simulation. *Clinical Simulation in Nursing*, 6(5), e177–e184.

Hamilton, N.A., Kieninger, A.N., Woodhouse, J., Freeman, B.D., Murray, D., Klingensmith, M.E. (2011). Video review using a reliable evaluation metric improves team function in high-fidelity simulated trauma resuscitation. *Journal of Surgical Education,* 69(3), 428–431.

Heath, C., Hindmarsh, J., & Luff, P. (2010). *Video in qualitative research.* London: SAGE Publications Ltd.

Hofvendahl, J. (2006). Riskabla samtal – en analys av. potentiella faror i skolans kvarts- och utvecklingssamtal [Risky conversations – an analysis of potential risks in quarter of an hour and development conferences in schools]. Linköping University: Arbetsliv i omvandling [Working life in transition] 2006:1.

Jefferson, G. (1984). Transcript notation. In M. Atkinson & J. Heritage (Eds.), *Structures of social action* (pp. ix– xvi). New York: Cambridge University Press.

Johansson, E., Lindwall, O., Rystedt, H. (2017). Experiences, appearances, and interprofessional training: The instructional use of video in post-simulation debriefings. *International Journal of Computer Supported Collaborative Learning,* 12(1), p. 91–112.

Lindwall, O., Lymer, G. (2014). Inquiries of the body: Novice questions and the instructable observability of endodontic scenes. *Discourse Studies,* 16(2), 271–294.

Lindwall, O., Johansson, E., Ivarsson, J., Rystedt, H., & Reit, C. (2014). The use of video in dental education: Clinical reality addressed as practical matters of production, interpretation, and instruction. In M. Broth, E. Laurier & L. Mondada (Eds.), *Studies of video practices: Video at work* (pp. 161–180). Abingdon: Routledge.

McIlvenny, P. (2011). Video interventions in everyday life: Semiotic and spatial practices of embedded video as a therapeutic tool in reality TV parenting programmes. *Social Semiotics,* 21(2), 259–288.

Oxelmark, L., Nordahl Amorøe, T., Carlzon, L., Rystedt, H. (2017). Students' understanding of teamwork and professional roles after interprofessional simulation—a qualitative analysis. *Advances in Simulation,* 2(8). https://doi.org/10.1186/s41077-017-0041-6.

Rystedt, H., Reit, C., Johansson, E., Lindwall, O. (2013). Seeing through the dentist's eyes: Video-based clinical demonstrations in preclinical dental training. *Journal of Dental Education,* 77(12), 1629–1638.

Savoldelli, L.G., Naik, N.V., Park, S.J., Joo, J.H., Chow, J., R., Hamstra, J. (2006). Value of debriefing during simulated crisis management: Oral versus video-assisted oral feedback. *Anesthesiology,* 105(2), 279–285.

Steinwachs, B. (1992). How to facilitate a debriefing. *Simulation & Gaming,* 23(2), 186–195.

Waring, H. Z. (2014). Mentor invitations for reflection in post-observation conferences: Some preliminary considerations. *Applied Linguistics Review,* 5(1), 99–123.

7.4   Commentary

Peter Dieckmann
Copenhagen Academy for Medical Education and Simulation (CAMES)
Center for Human Resources, Capital Region of Denmark
Copenhagen, Denmark

Department for Clinical Medicine
University of Copenhagen
Copenhagen, Denmark

Department for Quality and Health Technology
University of Stavanger
Stavanger, Norway
e-mail: mail@peter-dieckmann.de

In the first subchapter (7.2) by *Madeleine Abrandt Dahlgren* and *Samuel Edelbring*, the authors empirically demonstrate how the interactions of debriefing participants is related to physical characteristics of the room, relevant social rules, and the individual perspective and abilities of the acting persons. For debriefers, people who design scenarios, or debriefing rooms for that matter, considering interactions can make a big difference. This chapter emphasizes how those involved tune into each other in their sayings and doings. It is not only the debriefer, who influences the dynamic in the debriefing, they tune into the experience of their learners and guide them differently, depending on the context. Having identified this dynamic, makes me even more curious to investigate, which influences impact these interactions, and how those influences interact with each other.

The point, that I found most interesting in the chapter lies in the discussion of the results and relates to the frame of reference that is used during the debriefing. Where a lot of the debriefing interactions seem to be based on the individual perspective, Madeleine and Samuel point our attention to the alternative to consider debriefing as a professional/disciplinary space. I like this view as it foregrounds the actual value of debriefing (and simulation in general). All those involved in simulation, including the debriefers, the participants, but also the authors and you as a reader engage in the activities of simulating, debriefing, writing, reading to make a difference for patients, their relatives, and those who care for and treat them. It is not about the individual perspective – debriefing is not a personal space, not a therapeutic experience to help the individual to deal with a problem, not a coaching experience to help the individual to develop, not a team-development experience to improve team dynamics – even if simulation could be used to achieve these aims, and maybe it is used in this sense in this way. But – in the vast majority the interactions involved belong to the professional, not the personal space. This insight is not only an abstract conceptualization, it has a direct impact on the interactions in simulation settings. Which challenge should be discussed to what extend? What action should be praised? Is it appropriate to use a laissez-faire approach during the debriefing, or is the algorithm approach better suited? Those decisions are taken, too often, I think, as if they belonged to personal space, for example, in terms of the preferences of those involved. It is, however, a matter of the disciplinary space – defined by the aim with which the simulation setting was established and in which the dynamics unfold. The personal space is important, but, in most cases, belongs somewhere else. Tax payers, who finance simulation activities at least to a large extend are interested in simulation as professional, not as personal space. This chapter helped me to see this much more clearly and describes impressively the many different interactions involved that need to be analysed.

In the second Sect. 7.3 *Elin Nordenström, Torben Nordahl Amorøe and Hans Rystedt* discuss the use of video recordings during debriefings. They unfold the complexity of using video to support the learning of participants. Their theoretical perspectives and empirical findings show in an impressive way that any study investigating the learning benefits of using video would need to take the detailed use of the video into account. In my perspective do the existing studies comparing debriefings in which video was used to those in which it was not take this complexity into account well enough and this chapter can help tremendously in identifying those differences that actually make a difference (Bateson). Elin, Torben, and Hans also point to a way of investigating the use of video in a detailed way. It is a lot of work but promises to generate insights that can help in creating learning opportunities in and with simulation.

Part III
Simulation Pedagogy Re-Visited

Chapter 8
Bodies in Simulation

Peter Dieckmann, Ericka Johnson, and Nick Hopwood

8.1 Designing and Enacting the Simulated Body

Peter Dieckmann
Copenhagen Academy for Medical Education and Simulation (CAMES)
Center for Human Resources, Capital Region of Denmark
Copenhagen, Denmark

Department of Clinical Medicine
University of Copenhagen
Copenhagen, Denmark

Department for Quality and Health Technology
University of Stavanger
Stavanger, Norway
e-mail: mail@peter-dieckmann.de

Ericka Johnson
Department of Thematic Studies
Linköping University
Linköping, Sweden
ericka.johnson@liu.se

P. Dieckmann (✉)
Copenhagen Academy for Medical Education and Simulation (CAMES), Center for Human Resources, Capital Region of Denmark, Copenhagen, Denmark

Department of Clinical Medicine, University of Copenhagen, Copenhagen, Denmark

Department for Quality and Health Technology, University of Stavanger, Stavanger, Norway
e-mail: mail@peter-dieckmann.de

E. Johnson
Department of Thematic Studies, Linköping University, Linköping, Sweden
e-mail: ericka.johnson@liu.se

N. Hopwood
University of Technology Sydney, Sydney, Australia

University of Stellenbosch, Stellenbosch, South Africa
e-mail: nick.hopwood@uts.edu.au

M. Abrandt Dahlgren et al. (eds.), *Interprofessional Simulation in Health Care*,
Professional and Practice-based Learning 26,
https://doi.org/10.1007/978-3-030-19542-7_8

175

Simulation as a social practice (Dieckmann et al. 2007) brings together people who are interacting with each other, the environment, a range of equipment; the simulator is part of this equipment. A lot has been written about this interplay between the different elements in such an actor network (Sayes 2014). The body of the simulator is an important part of this social practice. How it is perceived, how it is simulated, how the simulated body is interacted with is the focus of this chapter. We unfold how this perspective matters for interprofessional use of simulations and begin by setting the stage in more general terms.

Much attention is paid to theorise, conceptualise and investigate pedagogical practices in using simulations and how effective they are. Such simulation settings are also used extensively for research. Research about simulation, where the simulator as a device, the simulation as social practice, or the design and implementation of simulators and simulations are foregrounded as the object of research (Rystedt and Lindstrom 2001; Sorensen et al. 2017; Johnson 2004). Research with simulation, on the other hand, uses simulation as a research setting to investigate other research objects, including certain types of interactions during care processes (Haig et al. 2006; Kolbe et al. 2012; Raemer et al. 2016), medication labels and their use (Dieckmann et al. 2016), or organisational aspects of care. (Barsuk et al. 2005; Biddell et al. 2016; Nielsen et al. 2014; Patterson et al. 2013) Studies that investigate the educational effectiveness of simulation activities and how those activities support (or hinder) transfer of learning draw on both angles: research on and with simulation. A certain use of the simulator is analysed for the effects that this use has.

Much of the theoretical work about simulators tends to focus on the body, often in terms of an investigation of how closely the simulator represents the "actual human body". Quantitative studies perform comparative measurements of body parts (Schebesta et al. 2011, 2012, 2015), while conceptual papers try to describe criteria against which the simulator and the simulations in which it is used are measured and compared to clinical practice. This chapter foregrounds the body in simulation, making it the main topic of interest. We build on previous work in trying to link theoretical conceptualizations with simulation practice. We also discuss potential "side effects" that bodies, their construction, and use might have in various simulation settings (e.g. basic education, advanced training, research, or assessment). This foreground is relevant, as different professions and disciplines in healthcare relate to the body in different ways. These differences can be due to various demands and anatomical interests of different medical specialisations (e.g. vascular surgery, ear-nose- and throat medicine, gynecology, psychiatry). These different foci on the body, their different construction of the body will have an impact on how bodies are replicated in simulation. Those body parts seen as relevant for the simulation goal might be replicated with more precision and/or functionality. In the context of this book, which addresses interprofessional learning and research, these different relations to the body are relevant as members in training courses or research projects might pose very different requirements on body simulators. Interprofessional training of cases in the operation room can serve as a good example. There are several simulators that allow one to create relevant learning opportunities for surgery. These do typically not include a possibility to simulate other parts of the body besides those that are needed for the training of the surgeries in focus. On the other hand, simulators that are useful for training anaesthesia procedures often provide only rudimentary or no possibilities to simulate operations. As consequence, to create simulations that focus on collaborative aspects of a medical procedure requires to either combine different simulators, which makes the control of the scenarios likely very complex; or that one or more members of the team work with simulators that might address their specific learning needs in only rudimentary ways. For some learning goals this might not actually be a (significant) limitation, but whenever the actual manipulation of the body in simulation is relevant for the learning goals, the limitations of simulating the body might be relevant.

By unfolding the way that one might think about and construct the body in material-discursive practices, that is, in the sayings and doings of simulator training, we hope not only to deepen the theoretical conceptualization of bodies in their relation to simulation and interprofessional work. We believe that such an improved conceptualization will contribute to optimize simulation practice. To do this, we use the example of a fat-pad in a gynaecological simulator.

Consider this fictitious scene:

Helena, a 32 years old physician in specialist training to become a gynaecologist, enters the simulation room. Her simulation instructor for today, Mia, has, in what Mia calls the 'scenario briefing', told her about the patient she is to see. The patient has experienced discomfort in her lower abdomen for a couple of days now and Helena is supposed to examine her. She is supposed to do the bimanual exam, while at the same time comforting the patient. Mia tells her that the patient is quite obese, with a body mass index of 31. Mia also says that Helena should keep the patient's obesity in mind, as the medical student portraying the patient is not actually obese (Margrethe, the student, is 24 years old with a BMI of 20). Referring to her own body in gestures, Mia explains to Helena that her Margrethe will hold a gynaecological simulator between her legs.

When Helena enters the room, she takes in the scene. Lene, a member of the simulation team portraying the role of a nurse, greets her and tells her what she knows about the patient. Helena listens, while looking at her patient. The picture is a bit funny actually. The medical student, Helena does not know her name – she forgot to ask about that during the simulation briefing – is sitting on a bed, wearing a hospital gown on top of her own underwear. Somehow, she is draped with hospital blankets – their main purpose here is to drape the interface between Margrethe and the simulator. The simulator itself consists of a pelvic replica with female abstracted external and detailed internal anatomy. After getting the handover, Helena approaches her patient to hear about what brings her here. She learns that the patient is called Linda (Margrethe preferred to pick a different name than her own) and has had discomfort for four days. Helena begins to manually examine Linda. She feels a strange bump on the uterus and is trying to remember what this might be a sign of, when she suddenly realises that Linda asked her a question. Lene is watching and her ears tingle as she realizes that Linda's question had gone unanswered.

The example above shows that healthcare simulation involves, in most cases, at least two bodies. The body of the patient and the body of the healthcare professional treating the patient. In the case of the example the picture is more complex. Helena uses her own body to explain to Mia how the body of the patient will be constructed inside of the simulation. She also asks Helena to "play along" and to mentally (and emotionally?) translate Margrethe's body she will see, into a patient body that is supposed to look different from what the visual impression is (the patient Linda is assumed to have a different BMI than Margrethe, the student portraying the patient, actually has). The patient's body can be seen as composed by two different entities: Margrethe's human body in combination with the plastic part task trainer. The task trainer focuses different aspects of the anatomy to different degrees. The outer anatomy is not needed for the learning goal and thus abstracted much more than the internal anatomy, which is in focus of this specific simulator. Finally, there is Lene's body – just as it is. But Lene's role is to pretend to be a different person. Her role is to take back a bit of her expertise and only do as she is asked for.

In the following, we will unpack this fictitious example around two questions:

1. What is a simulator simulating when a simulator simulates a body?
2. What modes of thinking are used when simulations reconstitute the senses, actors and bodies involved in the medical practices which are worked with and adjusted?
3. What knowledge is needed and how do we get this knowledge to reproduce the patient body in a purposeful way?
4. How can the body be enrolled in simulation in a way that supports a meaningful interaction with the body in a simulation setting, be it for education, training, or research?

8.1.1   Considering Body

Before we can simulate a body, we need to ask: What is a body? And what is a valid body to simulate? These questions touch on issues of identity and subjectivity, in as much as they query which types of bodies we want to simulate and thereby use as the representation of a 'normal' body for the users of the simulator. The concept of "normal" brings with it the question what the "normal" body in a simulator should be. Should it be a healthy body or a pathologized body, and if the simulator is being designed to simulate a pathology, whether the rest of the body should be "healthy". But even when a simulator is designed to simulate a healthy body, the question of "normal" can be tricky. What does medicine mean by normal: Standard? Average? Ideal? Healthy? And at what age in the lifespan? What point in the reproductive cycle? A child? An adult? A body of reproductive age? Or very old? Which size should the body be? Overweight, which is pretty normal in some contexts? Or suggested healthy weight, which is an ideal of medicine? Some simulators are designed to specifically address particular categories of patients (e.g. those with burns, traumas), but when a simulator is being designed to address a standard body, our understanding of what is 'standard' and 'normal' deserves to be critically appraised (Johnson 2005; Johnson and Berner 2010; Prentice 2005; Laqueur 1990; Waldby 2000). This is not least because the simulator is going to be a materialization of that normal, and as such will be a physical ambassador for the values embedded in the normativity it represents.

Once one has addressed the sort of body one wants to simulate, there is another pressing question – How do we create knowledge about the body in order to be able to reproduce it? Here the simulator community has been working very hard to come to grips with concepts of validity, realism, fidelity and developing technological advances that can help reproduce the human body in a way that is realistic and can also be quantitatively validated (Schebesta et al. 2011, 2012, 2015). But we would like to spend a few pages thinking first about how we know what a body is, what our knowledge making practices afford us in terms of descriptions and impressions, and how these reflections could be applied to the collection of knowledge about bodies before that knowledge is then reproduced. Our thoughts here are directed at the methods used to know what body should be simulated, before the technological approaches begin to simulate it. Then, further on in the chapter, we will be talking about how the simulated, materialized bodies can be enrolled into simulations.

But first, some words about ways of knowing the body and some philosophical thoughts about the materiality of a body and bodies made material.

To discuss this, we are going to use the example of a removable fat pad that was made for a gynaecological simulator. This simulator (see Fig. 1.1) was designed to help teach the bimanual pelvic exam, that standard exam a woman encounters when she goes to the gynaecologist. It is the one used in the simulation described in the introduction. During the exam, the gynaecologist inserts two fingers into the woman's vagina and, using the other hand to press down from on top of the abdomen, feels the cervix, the uterus and the ovaries, both checking that all parts are there and in place, and if there are any unusual bumps or growths on them. The exam has several aspects that are interesting with regards to the body. First, it is difficult to teach, because it is hard for a teacher to know if the student is actually feeling what s/he is supposed to be touching. Everything is inside the body, impossible to see. There is also potential embarrassment for both the patient and, at times, for healthcare professionals as well – especially in the beginning of their professional devel-

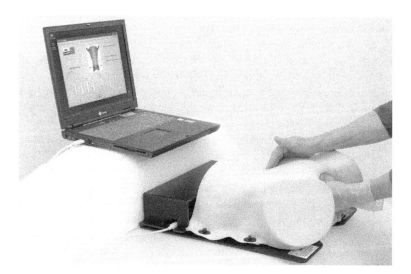

Fig. 1.1 Simulator for bimanual pelvic examination

opment, where their professionality is still in development. Finally, the exam is physically uncomfortable, for the woman being examined, but also for the examining physician as the different parts of the exam require some consideration about how one's body and hands are held in relation to the patient.

The example is also valuable in the context here, as the simulated procedure pinpoints cultural and historical ways of interacting with the body. The medical profession has long agonized over ways to create teaching settings that focus on certain aspects of the body in context, specifically decreasing the likelihood of other ways of interpreting the body (Henslin and Biggs 1971), which in the context of gynaecological exams also involves techniques to desexualize the patient-doctor relationship (Giuffre and Williams 2016).

The simulator addresses both that the exam could be uncomfortable to try on a patient, and that it is hard to know what the student is doing by providing a training opportunity without a real patient and by connecting the simulated internal organs to pressure sensors and a computer screen that could show if the student was touching where s/he is supposed to touch, and how hard. In this way, the simulator goes beyond a mere replication of the body. Some of the features of the body that become relevant in the context of activities performed with the body are emphasized, while others, not deemed relevant for the activity at hand, are neglected. While the key areas of the body that should be palpated are technologically enhanced, by including pressure sensors, the thighs and upper body of the simulator not replicated.

Ericka encountered this simulator when it was first purchased by a gynaecology department at a teaching hospital in Sweden (see Johnson 2008). The gynaecologists already had an existing training programme that used professional patients; women who volunteered to let students learn the exam on their bodies along with a gynaecologist teacher, and who were trained to tell the students what they were doing right and wrong, and how the exam felt on their bodies. These professional patients provided both a body (a "normal" body of sorts, even if it wasn't "normal", see Johnson forthcoming) and a subjectivity, that is, a patient who spoke, had a life history, and who could interact with the doctor during the exam. Hopwood et al. (2014) provide a detailed case study on this. We will return to the relationship of professional patients and simulator theory later in the chapter. In introducing the simulator to this teaching practice, the gynaecologists were responding to the dream of simulation, that the material artefact would be a sufficient stand-in to replace the human body.

The simulator had several different removable uteri, to simulate different "normal" bodies and a pathologized one, and it also came with a fat pad that could be inserted between the organs and the abdominal skin. One unfastened the skin, laid the fat pad over the organs, and then replaced the skin. This is because it is harder to feel parts of the anatomy, especially the ovaries, if a patient is obese and has a thick layer of fat between the gynaecologist's interior and exterior hand.

This fat pad, however, was the shape and thickness of a mouse pad, that silicon mat that we used to use with external computer mice back in the 1990s. This pad had a form that surprised many, who saw it for the first time, awaking questions about how such thin piece of silicon could simulate obesity.

The project involved doing in-depth interviews with the inventor and the designer of the simulator, so Ericka was able to ask about this fat pad. When Ericka asked the designer how the thin silicon was supposed to be an obese patient, she explained to her that fat in the body is at body temperature; it is warm. When it is that warm it is not very solid, and it has a tendency to move around almost (but not quite) like a liquid in parts of the body. She suggested Ericka thinks about a large cat lying on its back – much of the cat's fat will slide down of the apex of the stomach and gather along the cat's sides. Thus, when a patient is lying down on her back during the pelvic exam, as one does on the standard gynaecological exam tables (see Börjesson et al. 2016 for a norm critical analysis of these tables), the fat in her abdomen tends to slide downwards, off the peak of the stomach. When examining an obese patient's pelvic region, as the hands press up from inside and down from on top of the abdomen, even more of the fat in that area is gently pushed out of the way. Not all of it, of course, but quite a bit of it. Therefore, the 'thin' fat pad gives the feeling that a doctor would have when examining a much larger patient. The designer told Ericka:

> When you're going in, and someone's got that much fat, it will displace quite a lot […]. Whereas even though that silicon is very soft, it doesn't displace the same way. […] It's a matter of judging what is simulated, or how the simulation will equate with the real life.

We want to look closely at this quote and make two points, which we will do using two theoretical terms useful for knowing the body (or for knowing anything else in the world, for that matter).

The first point is that the designer was saying that the fat pad is simulating not the *actual body* of the patient, since it is not made of a gelatinous, almost liquid substance that moves out of the way and changes its behavior depending on temperature and position. In the most literal sense of the word, the fat pad is not a valid representation of body fat because it does not recreate the physical characteristics of fat. What the fat pad is simulating is the *phenomenon of feeling the body while examining an obese patient lying on her back*. The simulator becomes a valid representation of a specific practice, of a specific phenomenon of knowing patient obesity experienced by a doctor during a pelvic exam. To explain this better, we are going to use Donna Haraway's term, *apparatus of bodily knowledge*. The other point we want to make is that the fat – the body of the patient – is a relevant component of this 'body' being simulated, albeit one which is enrolled into the 'fat at body temperature during an exam' concept through a specific practice of knowing it. How we know it is constructed in the practice of examining the patient, but just because we mention it being constructed, doesn't mean there isn't a reality to the fat. It is there, pushing back. But to push back, we need to first feel it. We are speaking literally, but also metaphorically. To articulate that concept better, we are going to use Donna Haraway's term, *material-semiotic*.

Let us start with the concept of the *apparatus of bodily knowledge*. Donna Haraway uses this term to collect the different ideas, actors, things, and practices that together can be used to create knowledge about the world. In thinking through the fat pad, in asking how we can know what fat is, with this concept, we would consider the fat through time (being displaced), fat in a position (laying on one's back), fat inside a body (as part of the whole person), fat at body temperature (warm and of a certain viscosity), and fat between two hands (in this particular practice of knowing it). All of these together work as an apparatus of bodily knowledge, to produce what is then simulated as 'an obese patient'. Involved here, too, is the concept of the female reproductive tract as a valid object of medical interest, as a part of the anatomy that is both separate (The simulator starts at the navel and ends at the upper thigh – why do we draw those cuts? What makes that particular part of the anatomy of interest to gynecology? Answering this would draw on insights both about the history of the gynecological profession (Underman 2011; Bell 1979) and on critiques of how women's bodies have been medicalized in relation to their reproductive role (Dugdale 2000; Kline 2010; Maines 1999; Martin 1992)) and important enough to warrant a simulator. And an entire medical specialty, gynecology, for that matter. All of these values, practices and elements of the material world work together to create knowledge about an obese gynecological patient and a fat pad to simulate her.

Now a few words on the *material-semiotic*. This is a term that Donna Haraway introduced to feminist technoscience studies back in the 1990s to "highlight the object of knowledge as an active part of the apparatus of bodily production, without ever implying immediate presence of such objects or, what is the same thing, their final or unique determination of what can count as objective knowledge of a biomedical body at a particular historical juncture" (Haraway 1991: 208). Often, when simulators and their validity are spoken about, an ontologically discrete body is still the conceptual idea used to validate the simulator against measured bodies. Users and developers are still fixated on whether the anatomical measurement is right. But that isn't the right question to ask. If we understand the anatomy as a production of knowledge done through apparatuses of bodily knowledge, then we realize that there aren't ontologically discrete bodies, anywhere. Rather, there is a material-semiotic body. Simulator developers ought to ask how to figure out what the body is in that particular medical practice of knowing it, and then develop a simulator that simulates that practice, rather than the body as it can be quantified with different scanning or measurement techniques. If we reconceptualize our understanding of the body to be based on practice, or on phenomena of knowledge, as Barad would put it (Barad 2007), we could then develop methodological tools for approaching design that would be different. We would articulate and catch the phenomenon of knowing in practice. This practice would also emphasize the activity in which the simulator is used. There are, to some extent differences in the activities between the clinical setting (diagnosing and treating patients) and the simulation setting (learning to diagnose and treat patients, optimizing diagnosis and treatment processes, testing the abilities to diagnose and treat patients. etc.). And these would be more easily addressed through methods that measured or otherwise captured practices of knowing the body, instead of concentrating on context-insensitive physical measurements of the body.

The material of the material-semiotic means that the world pushes back. It is referring to the material component of knowledge objects. The semiotic is the other part of the actor, the tropes, discourses, models – or mental images and the way we have been taught by physical representations, like simulators, which are entangled with the world as we make sense of it, as we make knowledge about it. This is the reason why it is so important to think through our modelling practices, because the results of those practices have long reaching effects. But it is also why it is important to think through our knowledge making practices in the first place. As we make knowledge in very specific practices, we are making contextualized and specific, contingent knowledges. Passing these off as standard truths, ontologically divorced from practice, is misrepresenting them to ourselves, and to others. Instead, our knowledge (of in this case an obese abdomen) is *situated*, is produced through particular examination practices and through particular material constellations of bodies, tables, hands… these must be considered in the way we represent fat (Johnson 2015). We would suggest that the simulator designer was aware of this. She articulated it when she told Ericka: "It's a matter of judging what is simulated, or how the simulation will equate with the real life". She was working within a discursive framework that demanded quantifiable descriptions of the anatomy, but she was thinking about practice, where adjustments to the material of the simulator are frequent, as are adjustments of the instructions around how to use the simulator and how to interpret its physicality, and adjustments of how a given scenario is implemented for a specific user.

Thinking about simulators and the validity of their body models is particularly important as long as one also considers the possibility that simulators will be teaching users specific skills, as if the simulators themselves had the agency to do so. This understanding of agency, however, builds on a common tendency to attribute agency to people (and in the simulator example, things) as if agency were a possession which could be actioned. But Lucy Suchman's work with computer interfaces (Suchman 2007) suggests instead that agency be imagined as relational and distributed across the human machine divide, enacted through practice. Her writings force questions about where we create a division between the human and the machine, why, and how those divisions require work to be done and maintained. She is also keen to point out that these divisions are asymmetrical and question the political and power structures involved in them. We find her discussions so useful and inspiring for how I could respond to concerns about the agency of the simulators in teaching situations. If, following Suchman, one reconsiders agency along the same lines as one reconsiders objective knowledge of bodily anatomies, and instead thinks of agency as a relational practice between the material artefact and the user, then agency becomes something not located in the person (or simulator) creating knowledge, but in the relational practices with the materiality of the examined body that unfold in activities of learning, doing research, testing, etc. (see chapter 5b this volume).

Adjustments to the relational practice can be made in different areas: In the simulator's material body, b) software controlling the simulator displaying physiology and c) the practice implemented in the scenarios. To make any training situation comparable, test situations fair, and not to overload students (and simulation educators) with too much complexity, many scenarios might actually fall short to capture the complexity of care – not (only) in terms of the simulation of the (patho-)physiology of the patient, but also with regards to how the simulator body is approached.

(Miranda 2016, p. 40) Such interactions might be programmed into controlling software or defined in checklists and observation sheets. Those represent idealized practices as "universal technologies" (Berg and Timmermans after Miranda, 2016, p. 41) or might be called "universal approaches". They focus on the practice stripped of context factors and were questioned (Soffer 2015). When implemented in simulation or clinical practice approaches to the body, interaction with the patient will need to be adapted to the context again. Work as imagined is not equal to work as done (Hollnagel 2014, 2017).

The software controlling the simulator can be seen as part of the body in manikin-based simulators. It represents the physiological changes. Especially in the software, but also in the hardware adjustments are made frequently to the "standard body" to cater for local flavors of practice, to adjust to target groups, or learning goals – to name but a few of the criteria that crave adjustments. (Hirsch et al. 2016) Miranda (2016) describes adjustments made to pre-programmed scenarios controlling the physiology of the patient. Many adjustments can be found to simulation bodies to enhance them with regards to the way they are used: lights were placed under the skin of the simulator to indicate a rush on the thorax of the patient. Another simulation center, having employed an engineer and working a lot with cardiologists, "pimped" their simulator with a whole array of connectors for 12-lead ECGs so that the simulator body was purposefully enhanced to allow for training scenarios relevant in the practice, where the simulator was used. We call such elements "y elements" and explain them in the following paragraph. A mix of learning needs and wishes, technical understanding, nerdy playfulness and many other things will influence how the simulator body is seen, worked with and adjusted.

8.1.2 Considering Simulating the Body

The discussion so far has established that the body is constructed in the context of activities. Simulating this body means to replicate phenomena that are relevant for the aim of the simulator use. Not all can be simulated, for example due to technical limitations. Not all should be simulated, for example to not end in the same level of complexity (and vulnerability) as with a human being. It depends on the activity in which the simulator is encountered which part its materiality plays in the relational practices.

Let us pick up on the designer's word above of the equation, which resonates with previous work (Dieckmann 2009). The simulator does not replicate some features of a human body but adds other features not found in the human body. Let us term the "missing parts" as x and the added parts as "y". Then we can consider the following formula: Simulator Body = (Human Body − x) + y. This equation can be based on the physical characteristics of the simulated and the simulating body. It can also be based on the phenomena that are made possible by the material involved (fat in the case of the human, silicon in the case of the simulator). It is a case of the material and the discursive becoming one phenomenon of knowledge, as Barad (2007) would put it. Both variables in the equation are interesting to investigate. In many contexts, attempts are made to minimize x in the equation, resulting in surprisingly realistic replica of bodies and their parts – in art (https://artmap.com/arken/exhibi-tion/gosh-is-it-alive-2017) and in robotics (https://www.youtube.com/watch?v=ITLyfGqua6A). This speaks to the age-old human fascination of replicat-ing the human body as closely as possible. In the context of (interprofessional) training, minimizing x is often seen as an implicit (or explicit) quality criterion for the value of the simulator. The y elements can be seen as purposeful changes to characteristics of the simulated body that aim to enhance how it supports learning or other purposes of using the simulator. This can be sensors, as mentioned, or color coding of anatomical structures, building in cameras on the inside of the simulator to provide a possibility to have a view inside, or to make the simulator transparent to fulfil the same function.

One aspect that simulation should support is the embodiment of competence. Miranda (2016) describes how an experienced nurse participating in her study describes the embodiment of her competences in interacting with patient bodies: "You learn to pick up on these things over time. Smelling an infected wound, hear-ing a slight rattle in the someone's breathing, feeling a feverish body….This isn't something that you are able to do on the first day, or maybe even in the first year. But the more patients your care for, the better you become at noticing these different things […] I have to admit that most of the time I don't even think about it anymore. […] but I think it makes me a better nurse in some ways. "(Miranda 2016) Miranda's example emphasizes the variety of senses involved in the embodiment. Lahlou describes this embodiment as happening through experiences: sense impressions, considerations, reflections, etc. over time. Each case is slightly different, forming the basis for building up one's own embodied abilities (Lahlou 2017).

We offer a framework of three different modes of thinking about reality and thus the simulators' reality to investigate the correspondence between relational prac-tices in clinical and environments and those in simulation-based settings. These modes address how simulation can support the embodiment of competences. The *physical mode of thinking* describes those features (and only those features) that can be measured in cm, gram, seconds – or any derivations of these dimensions. The measurement of body parts, their weight, the light wavelengths reflected from the simulators skin, the timely characteristics of changes in electrical resistance patterns at the monitoring contacts of the simulator. In the case of the gynecological simula-tor, for example, this would include the way the pressure sensor wires were strung behind the uterus and up to the computer and the way they registered and then dis-played pressure on the computer screen. The *semantical mode of thinking* describes the meaning that is enabled via the physical characteristics of the simulator. This meaning is context dependent, influenced by culture, work procedures, learned focus points, motivations, norms, values, and beliefs. Some participants will form a meaning of the simulator body that is shared with others. They understand the simu-lator as representing a certain disease, for example. An investigation of the simula-tor body leads them to the same conclusion about what is simulated. Other participants, however, might draw a different conclusion from the same physical constellation of the body. Some elements for their understanding are not simulated, for example. Without the clinical impression of the patient's temperature it might be hard for them to form an understanding of the patient simulated (see chapter 4b this volume). In the case of the gynecological simulator, the wiring allowed for an American bimanual exam but hindered the practice of flipping back the uterus when doing a Swedish style bimanual exam, which displayed the semantic aspect of how a uterus' anatomy was understood and modelled and how this was related to culturally specific practices (Johnson 2008). Finally, there is the *phenomenal mode of thinking* that looks at the human experience in real life and in the simulation. How do those involved experience the interactions in the situation? Which feelings, emotions, perceptions, thoughts etc. are involved in this experience. In the fictional scenario at the beginning of this chapter, the phenomenal mode is represented by the person giving voice and personality to the simulation, Margrethe. In the actual gynecological teaching that Ericka observed in Sweden, the phenomenal mode was accentuated by the use of professional patients who volunteered to let their bodies be examined by students.

Participants can choose, for example, to concentrate on the features of the simulator body that is in line with the learning goals and with their clinical experience. They can also choose to concentrate on technical imperfections, inconsistent use of the simulator. In case of the gynecological simulator, would learners in the US experience the simulator as matching their practice, where their Swedish colleagues might be confused as the simulator does not allow them to enact an important part of their practice.

8.1.3   Simulating Various Bodies

These modes of thinking about simulation realism, described in the last paragraph, bring us back to the notion of "normal". When looking through exhibition areas and catalogues of simulation manufacturers, there is (necessarily) a limited range of bodies offered – many as close to the "real human" body as possible. There are, however, interesting exceptions to this rule, where the simulator focused on the functional aspect of the task to be learned – helping in the delivery process and to prevent post-partum hemorrhage for birthing simulators, for example. Based on considerations of cultural norms that would not support the detailed replication of the body, and especially its sex organs, does the Mamanatalie simulator specifically work with a very abstracted form of a part of the female body (https://www.laerdal. com/dk/products/simulation-training/obstetrics-paediatrics/mamanatalie/). Being built to support birthing in low income countries there were also considerations to make the simulator durable and usable in outside settings (Sundén 2010). As the simulator works with actual liquids to simulate blood, easy cleaning was another design feature implemented. The simulator is a good example for how the different modes of thinking about realism can play together. The simulator provides the salient cues that are needed to experience relevant phenomena in the context of a very sharply defined situation. It does so with very "unrealistic" materials – but those support the use of the simulator, not the least in regard to cultural norms. This example shows that many different angles are relevant, when considering how a simulator is designed. The different stakeholders construct its reality in their own way: the designers might think of the moving parts or material specifications; the educators about how well key issues of actual physiology are represented in the simulator and how easy it is to control; some stakeholders might consider how many of the ingredients of the simulator can be recycled and so on. Our fictional example also shows how humans can engage purposefully in the simulation, engaging into a "fiction contract" (Dieckmann et al. 2007; Eco 1994) that makes it possible for them to believe in a scenario, where some of the triggers of the simulator would not support a realistic impression on a physical basis.

Another issue in the combination of the simulated body – both in terms of its material aspects and the simulated processes concerns simulations around "irregular" cases. Consider simulations of transgender people. In male to female transgender patients, who are under hormone therapy, some prostate laboratory findings need to be interpreted differently than in male patients without hormone therapy. (Greene et al. 2014, 2017; Roberts et al. 2014) The same result of an investigation needs to be interpreted differently in these patients. These scenarios also create a challenge beyond the physiological level. Consider a patient with a male body, who identifies as female, uses female pronouns, and carries a female name. For simulation participants this might be confusing, as it might not be obvious for them, whether the scenario is meant to involve a patient with these characteristics (a relatively rare event), or whether the simulation team made a consistency error in the design or running of the scenario (a relatively frequent event). In addition, as many simulators represent a male body, but are often used in scenarios where the simulator is supposed to be a female patient, participants are not necessarily tuned into really considering the anatomy of the patient, if the scenario does not directly involve anatomy-related issues. Here the limitations of the simulator and the way that it is used actually make it more difficult to cover the learning around "nonstandard" patients. We speculate that human simulators might have an advantage here over manikin-based simulators in sensitizing to such issues. It is easier to find out whether the inconsistency is a part of the scenario, or a consistency error.

As a further example, Miranda (2016) describes an episode where nursing students had challenges in learning to perform chest compressions. In the situation described, the students rather frequently broke the chest compartment of the simulator. Such a damage corresponds actually to healthcare practice, where up to one third of adult patients experience rib fractures during resuscitation (Hoke and Chamberlain 2004). In the learning situation, however, the students actually decreased the force used during compressions as they were afraid of breaking the training device. Here the physical aspects of the simulation correspond to human patients, but the experience of the situation seems to be different with possible negative effects on the application of what was learned in training. There was also a very practical consequence described in the setting. In cases when the simulator broke during the automated exercise in which the nursing students encountered it, they would not get the paper-based certificate needed. It would take additional work to obtain the paper needed – potentially having to redo the session, resulting in potential delays in their study progress.

8.1.4   Conclusion

Returning to the fictitious gynecological simulation presented at the beginning of this chapter, we would like to conclude with a few words about simulated bodies and simulations of practice on them. The first perspective perhaps being most relevant for those who design simulators and the second for those who use them in educational or other settings. As we pointed out above, not only the physical body is relevant here, but also how it – and the patient embodied in that body – is interacted with, thought of, felt about in active interaction with it. The *material-semiotic* body as known through the exams and the *apparatus of bodily knowledge* produces important, contingent aspects of anatomy-medical practice to consider when designing simulators. Differences between the body in simulation and the body in clinical practice can be so small that they are not noticeable, but it is useful to remember that the 'body in clinical practice' is the smallest ontological unit possible of knowing (Barad 2007). Any questions of validity of fidelity are asked to the body as a knowledge phenomenon.

If differences between the patient body in clinical practice and the body in simulation are noticeable they can contribute to building the" wrong" embodied abilities: the finger tips are calibrated to" unrealistic" tissues characteristics; the procedural memory remembers wrong steps, makes up steps that should not be there, or forgets steps in a procedure. Noticeable differences, however can also be used to reflect upon practice: what do the confused finger tips tell a learner about the construction of the body and diagnostic and intervention considerations? What would happen if a step would be added to a procedure, another being left out? Such differences can become obvious when the clinical impression is simulated, which is such a vital part of clinical practice:" Sliding down a thumb across the top of a patient's hand to get a feel for the quality of the veins, while gently holding it for comfort, or holding a patient's hand on the top of her chest to soothe her anxiety while getting a feel for the quality, depths, and evenness of her breathing" (Soffer 2015). The three modes of thinking about simulators' reality can improve the conceptualization of differences between the simulator and the body it simulates and can also be used to investigate the how simulators might be used to replicate some of these many functions of interacting with the body: *the physical mode* of thinking which is often measured in quantitative aspects of the simulator and its representation of patient bodies; *the semantical mode* of thinking, which considers the cultural, social and medical specialist communities of practice, and their unique understandings of medicine and the body; and *the phenomenal mode* of thinking, which gives considered attention to the experiential elements of simulations.

By shifting the learning from the patient body to the simulator body, one gets a set of features including the possibility for "endless training" in an environment, that does not endanger patients. The different ways of constructing the body in the interaction between its purpose and its users can provide some depths to the discussion of how simulators can be built and used in the context of interprofessional learning. The different practices of healthcare in the different disciplines and professions practice the body, feel the body, interact with the body in different ways.

These differences can be interesting learning opportunities, when discovered and discussed. The understanding of these differences can help also to design simulation scenarios and debriefings that are useful for learners of different backgrounds.

References

Barad, K. (2007). *Meeting the universe half-way*. Durham: Duke University Press.
Barsuk, D., Ziv, A., Lin, G., Blumenfeld, A., Rubin, O., Keidan, I., et al. (2005). Using advanced simulation for recognition and correction of gaps in airway and breathing management skills in prehospital trauma care. *Anesthesia Analgesia, 100*(3), 803–809. doi:https://doi.org/10.1213/01.ANE.0000143390.11746.CF.
Bell, S. (1979). Political gynecology: Gynecological imperialism and the politics of self-help. *Science for the People*, 11, 8–14.
Biddell, E. A., Vandersall, B. L., Bailes, S. A., Estephan, S. A., Ferrara, L. A., Nagy, K. M., et al. (2016). Use of simulation to gauge preparedness for ebola at a free-standing children's hospital. *Simulation in Healthcare, 11*(2), 94–99. doi:https://doi.org/10.1097/SIH.0000000000000134.
Börjesson, E., Isaksson, A., Ilstedt, S. & Ehrnberger, K. (2016)." Visualizing gender – norm-critical design and innovation". In G. A. Alsos, U. Hytti & E. Ljunggren (Eds.). *Research handbook on gender and innovation*. London: Edward Elgar Publishing Limited.
Dieckmann, P. (2009). Simulation settings for learning in acute medical care. In P. Dieckmann (Ed.), *Using simulation for education, training and research* (pp. 40–138). Lengerich: Pabst.
Dieckmann, P., Gaba, D., Rall, M. (2007). Deepening the theoretical foundations of patient simulation as social practice. *Simulation in Healthcare, 2*(3), 183–193. doi:https://doi.org/10.1097/SIH.0b013e3180f637f5.
Dieckmann, P., Clemmensen, M. H., Sorensen, T. K., Kunstek, P., Hellebek, A. (2016). Identifying facilitators and barriers for patient safety in a medicine label design system using patient simulation and interviews. *Journal of Patient Safety, 12*(4), 210–222. doi:https://doi.org/10.1097/PTS.0000000000000109.
Dugdale, A., (2000). Materiality: Juggling Sameness and Difference. In J. Law & J. Hassard (Eds.), *Actor network theory and after* (pp. 113–135). Oxford: Blackwell.
Eco, U. (1994). *Six walks in the fictional woods*. Cambridge, MA: Harvard University Press.
Greene, R. E., Garment, A. R., Avery, A., Fullerton, C. (2014). Transgender history taking through simulation activity. *Medical Education, 48*(5), 531–532. doi:https://doi.org/10.1111/medu.12439.
Greene, R. E., Hanley, K., Cook, T. E., Gillespie, C., Zabar, S. (2017). Meeting the primary care needs of transgender patients through simulation. *Journal of*

Graduate Medical Education, 9(3), 380–381. doi:https://doi.org/10.4300/JGME-D-16-00770.1.

Giuffre, P. A., & Williams, C. L. (2016). Not just bodies. Strategies for desexualizing the physical examination of patients. *Gender & Society,* 14(2), 457–482.

Haig, K. M., Sutton, S., Whittington, J. (2006). SBAR: A shared mental model for improving communication between clinicians. *Joint Commission Journal on Quality and Patient Safety,* 32(3), 167–175.

Haraway, D. (1991). *Simians, cyborgs, and women. The reinvention of nature.* London: Free Association Books.

Henslin, J. M., & Biggs, M. A., (1971). Dramatical desexualization: The sociology of the vaginal examination. In J. M. Henslin (Ed.), *Studies in the sociology of sex* (pp. 243–272). New York: Appleton-Century-Crofts.

Hirsch, J., Generoso, J. R., Latoures, R., Acar, Y., Fidler, R. L. (2016). Simulation manikin modifications for high-fidelity training of advanced airway procedures. *A Case Rep, 6*(9), 268–271. doi:https://doi.org/10.1213/XAA.0000000000000278.

Hoke, R. S., & Chamberlain, D. (2004). Skeletal chest injuries secondary to cardiopulmonary resuscitation. *Resuscitation, 63*(3), 327–338. doi:https://doi.org/10.1016/j.resuscitation.2004.05.019.

Hollnagel, E. (2014). *Safety-I and safety-II: the past and future of safety management.* Farnham: Ashgate Publishing Company.

Hollnagel, E. (2017). *Safety-II in practice: developing the resilience potentials.* Abingdon: Routledge.

Hopwood, N., Abrandt Dahlgren, M., & Siwe, K. (2014). Developing professional responsibility in medicine: A sociomaterial curriculum. In T. Fenwick & M. Nerland (Eds.), *Reconceptualising professional learning: Sociomaterial knowledges, practices, and responsibilities* (pp. 171–183). London: Routledge.

Johnson, E. (2004). *Situating Simulators: The integration of simulations in medical Practice.* Lund: Arkiv (PhD Dissertation).

Johnson, E. (2005). The Ghost of Anatomies Past: Simulating the one-sex body in modern medical training. *Feminist Theory,* 6(2), 141–59.

Johnson, E. (2008). Simulating medical patients and practices: Bodies and the construction of valid medical simulators. *Body and Society,* 14(3), 105–128.

Johnson, E. (2015). Intra-face. A Poem. *European Journal of Women's Studies* 22(3), 356–357.

Johnson, E. (forthcoming). *Refracting through technologies. Seeing and untangling bodies, medical technologies and discourses.* Routledge.

Johnson, E. & B. Berner (Eds.), (2010). *Technology and medical practices. Blood, guts and machines.* Farnham: Ashgate.

Kline, W. (2010). *Bodies of knowledge: Sexuality, reproduction, and women's health in the second wave.* Chicago: University of Chicago Press.

Kolbe, M., Burtscher, M. J., Wacker, J., Grande, B., Nohynkova, R., Manser, T., Grote, G. (2012). Speaking up is related to better team performance in simulated anesthesia inductions: An observational study. *Anesthesia Analgesia, 115*(5), 1099–1108. doi:https://doi.org/10.1213/ANE.0b013e318269cd32.

Lahlou, S. (2017). *Installation theory. The societal construction and regulation of behaviour.* Cambridge: Cambridge University Press.

Laqueur, T. (1990). *Making sex: Body and gender from the greeks to freud.* London: Harvard University Press.

Maines, R., (1999). *The technology of orgasm.* Baltimore: John Hopkins University Press.

Martin, E. (1992). *The woman in the body: A cultural analysis of reproduction.* Boston: Beacon Press.

Nielsen, D. S., Dieckmann, P., Mohr, M., Mitchell, A. U., Ostergaard, D. (2014). Augmenting health care failure modes and effects analysis with simulation. *Simulation in Healthcare, 9*(1), 48–55. doi:https://doi.org/10.1097/SIH.0b013e3182a3defd.

Patterson, M. D., Geis, G. L., Falcone, R. A., LeMaster, T., Wears, R. L. (2013). In situ simulation: Detection of safety threats and teamwork training in a high risk emergency department. *BMJ Qual Saf, 22*(6), 468–477. doi:https://doi.org/10.1136/bmjqs-2012-000942.

Prentice, R., (2005). The anatomy of surgical simulation: the mutual articulation of bodies in and through the machine. *Social Studies of Science* 35(6), 837–66.

Raemer, D. B., Kolbe, M., Minehart, R. D., Rudolph, J. W., Pian-Smith, M. C. (2016). Improving anesthesiologists' ability to speak up in the operating room: A randomized controlled experiment of a simulation-based intervention and a qualitative analysis of hurdles and enablers. *Academic Medicine, 91*(4), 530–539. doi:https://doi.org/10.1097/ACM.0000000000001033.

Roberts, T. K., Kraft, C. S., French, D., Ji, W., Wu, A. H., Tangpricha, V., Fantz, C. R. (2014). Interpreting laboratory results in transgender patients on hormone therapy. *American Journal of Medicine, 127*(2), 159–162. doi:https://doi.org/10.1016/j.amjmed.2013.10.009.

Rystedt, H., Lindstrom, B. (2001). Introducing simulation technologies in nurse education: A nursing practice perspective. *Nurse Education in Pracicet, 1*(3), 134–141. doi:https://doi.org/10.1054/nepr.2001.0022.

Sayes, E. (2014). Actor-Network Theory and methodology: Just what does it mean to say that nonhumans have agency? *Social Studies of Science, 44*(1), 134–149. doi:https://doi.org/10.1177/0306312713511867.

Schebesta, K., Hupfl, M., Ringl, H., Machata, A. M., Chiari, A., Kimberger, O. (2011). A comparison of paediatric airway anatomy with the SimBaby high-fidelity patient simulator. *Resuscitation, 82*(4), 468–472. doi:https://doi.org/10.1016/j.resuscitation.2010.12.001.

Schebesta, K., Hupfl, M., Rossler, B., Ringl, H., Muller, M. P., Kimberger, O. (2012). Degrees of reality: Airway anatomy of high-fidelity human patient simulators and airway trainers. *Anesthesiology, 116*(6), 1204–1209. doi:https://doi.org/10.1097/ALN.0b013e318254cf41.

Schebesta, K., Spreitzgrabner, G., Horner, E., Hupfl, M., Kimberger, O., Rossler, B. (2015). Validity and fidelity of the upper airway in two high-fidelity patient simulators. *Minerva Anestesiology, 81*(1), 12–18.

Miranda, A. K. B. (2016). *Caring for plastic: An ethnography of simulation-based training in nursing education.* København: DPU, Aarhus Universitet.

Soffer, A. K. B. (2015). Replacing and representing patients: Professional feelings and plastic body replicas in nursing education. *Emotion, Space and Society*, 16, 11–18.

Sorensen, J. L., Ostergaard, D., LeBlanc, V., Ottesen, B., Konge, L., Dieckmann, P., Van der Vleuten, C. (2017). Design of simulation-based medical education and advantages and disadvantages of in situ simulation versus off-site simulation. *BMC Medical Education, 17*(1). doi:https://doi.org/10.1186/s12909-016-0838-3.

Suchman, L. (2007). *Human machine reconfigurations. Plans and situated actions second edition.* Cambridge: Cambridge University Press.

Sundén, J. (2010). Blonde birth machines: Medical simulation, techno-corporeality and posthuman feminism. In E. Johnson & B. Berner (Eds.), *Technology and medical practices. Blood, guts and machines* (pp. 97–117). Farnham: Ashgate.

Underman, K. (2011). "It's the knowledge that puts you in control": The embodied labor of gynecological educators. *Gender & Society*, 25(4), 431–450.

Waldby, C. (2000). *The visible human project: Informatic bodies and posthuman medicine.* New York: Routledge.

8.2   Commentary

8.2.1   Do Simulators Actually Simulate Bodies? Provocations, Problems and Prospects

Nick Hopwood
University of Technology Sydney
Sydney, Australia

University of Stellenbosch
Stellenbosch, South Africa
e-mail: nick.hopwood@uts.edu.au

What is a simulator simulating when a simulator simulates a body? Dieckmann and Johnson's response is charged with welcome disruptions that recast connected questions about modes of thinking, knowledge, and pedagogy. In these reflections I address arguments made within or sparked by their writing, relishing the provocations that result, problematizations they draw to our attention, and prospects that emerge if we follow Dieckmann and Johnson's lines of thinking.

8.2.1.1 Provocations

Asking "What is a simulator simulating when a simulator simulates a body?" is itself a provocation. It implies that the answer is not simply, "a body". Many have taken up the obvious but narrow meaning of this question, fixating on 'whether the anatomical measurement is right'. What else could a medical simulator simulate, other than a body, or at least part of a body? Part of Dieckmann and Johnson's answer is that a simulator simulates different kinds of bodies – healthy, pathological, perhaps gendered (see below). We also learn how simulators simulate sensations of contact with the body – as with the surprisingly thin fat pad that "replicates" feelings of touching an obese patient. There is something profoundly unsettling in the way this question is asked and answered. Such unsettling is, in my view, overdue, necessary, and productive.A second provocation is not announced as such in the text, but rather flows from it. There is a sense from the examples of fat pads and of a pelvic simulator in combination with a student actor (Margrethe/Linda), that the simulators don't simulate 'real' bodies at all. They simulate bodies that never actually exist. Fakes. They simulate ideas, or perhaps (problematic) ideals. Maybe they are not simulations at all, but simulacra, in the way Baudrillard (1981, 1983) would have us understand the term. Theme parks enchant us with replicas of a "Wild West" that never existed. Maybe what makes simulators interesting and valuable is their capacity to represent or imitate bodies in ways that are not tied to the 'real' body (Hopwood 2017). Elsewhere in this book readers can encounter simulators as substitutes for the 'undying body' (Anh and Rimpiläinen: "The simulation exercise always has a happy ending"), and here in Chap. 8 we find the nameless body, the fractured body (half real person, half plastic assemblage), the easy-to-clean body, and simulations (no! simulacra) of the non-existing "norma" body.

8.2.1.2 Problems

Dieckmann and Johnson discuss what the "side effects" that bodies and their use might have in simulation. Some of these concern ways in which simulators or simulations can uphold problematic notions of the body. There is no such thing as a standard patient, yet simulators are often based in the fiction of the standard. There is no such thing as a normal patient, yet simulators are often based in the fiction of the norm. Simulacra masquerading as simulations can be dangerous. The authors are not the first to highlight the simulator as "physical ambassador for the values embedded in the normativity it represents", adding to the conceptual tools at our disposal to grapple with these issues by focusing on contextualised, specific and contingent knowledges and modes of thinking, for example. They question what the simulator embodies or implies about size, lifespan, age, and gender, voicing important concerns about how simulators and people around them can incorporate gender fluidity and ambiguity. When and how do simulators erase variation in relation to bodies being differently abled/disabled, coloured, and even classed (surely class inscribes itself in and on the body)? "Real" bodies disappear, and the act of erasure disappears with them.

There are traces of other side-effects too. Is there a current in Dieckman and Johnson's argument that a side-effect of simulators is that students, educators and researchers get side-tracked? Does the tail wag the dog? Does the quest for authenticity in the artefact divert our gaze from what actually matters – practices? The example of bimanual exams in America and Sweden speaks powerfully to this. Do technological affordances hold us in a distracting physical mode of thinking, when other modes also demand our attention? Does our desire to replace human bodies (because they can feel pain, be injured, etc.) side-track us into a desire to re-produce them, rather than put in place more creative, dare I say it, unrealistic alternatives?

8.2.1.3 Prospects

Which leads me to prospects that the authors offer us directly and otherwise. By letting go of the ontologically discrete body, Dieckmann and Johnson offer alternative ways of understanding simulators and simulations, showing the relevance of Haraway's concept of the apparatus of bodily knowledge, in which bodies push back, provided, of course we feel them. This, and Haraway's notion of the material-semiotic underpin their framework of three modes of thinking – physical, semantic and phenomenal – through which we can think in more sophisticated ways about bodies and simulation.

The chapter offers an equation: Simulator Body = (Human Body – x) + y (where x refers to the 'missing parts' and y refers to 'added parts'). I would like to expand on this through the metaphor of the topological map. A topological map is a simplified representation of selected parts of the world. Many readers will be familiar with using them to navigate urban underground rail networks. Harry Beck's representation of London's Tube network caught on as an effective principle in many cities around the world. What makes them so useful, and what relevance do they have to do with simulated bodies?

Topological maps work because of what they take out, not just what they include. Mapping transport networks is not a question of reducing "x" to the smallest value possible, rather the opposite: taking out all that is superfluous to the practice of navigating from one place to another (for example, scale, distance, compass direction). Dieckmann and Johnson describe the occupation of many in simulation with "minimising x", and tantalise us with a not-quite-stated prospect that perhaps the reverse is true. Isn't what simulators don't reproduce important as a productive force rather than imitative failing?

What about the "+y"? Isn't what makes simulators so exciting their capacity to go beyond real bodies? Why does the miracle of simulation – you can always bring the body back to life – translate into practices where the patient is never allowed to die (see Chap. 5)? The fantastic possibilities of pausing, rewinding, and trying again are fantastical – but potentially pedagogically powerful.

8.2.1.4 Concluding Remarks: Fiction

A synoptic way of thinking about Dieckman and Johnson's piece is in terms of fiction. They mention the "fiction contract" in which participants tolerate realism and ruptures with it. What other fictions are we alerted to? Explicitly, the authors confront us with the fiction of the standard or normal body and the fiction of the agentic simulator – as if it simulates anything by itself. On my reading, we also encounter the fiction of simulation over simulacrum, and the fiction of the diminishing "x". Perhaps a lesson from this chapter is that provocations, problematisations and prospects in understanding simulation might be further advanced if we embrace fictional worlds of fantasy and the unreal, rather than fixating on the real.

References

Baudrillard, J. (1981). *Simulacra and simulation*. Ann Arbor: University of Michigan Press.

Baudrillard, J. (1983). *Simulations*. New York: Semiotext[e].

Hopwood, N. (2017). Practice architectures of simulation pedagogy: From fidelity to transformation. In K. Mahon, S. Francisco, & S. Kemmis (Eds.), *Exploring education and professional practice: Through the lens of practice architectures* (pp. 63–81). Dordrecht: Springer.

Chapter 9
Advancing Simulation Pedagogy and Research

Hans Rystedt, Madeleine Abrandt Dahlgren, Li Felländer-Tsai, and Sofia Nyström

9.1 Introduction

An overall conclusion from prior research on interprofessional learning is that simulation could be beneficial for the development of competencies needed for successful teamwork. However, the lack of attention to the practice of simulation itself and how people are learning together, creates a knowledge gap which the chapters in this book contribute to bridge by taking the "turn to practice" seriously. This approach is especially important for research on simulation-based interprofessional training, since it implies an analytical focus on the different roles and responsibilities permeating teamwork; the significance of the ways in which briefing, scenario and debriefing are designed, and how various perspectives and professional concerns are played out and negotiated in simulation-based learning.

In this final chapter, we will first turn to the empirical findings and draw conclusions on what these findings add to previous research on interprofessional simulation. Secondly, we will discuss the methodological contributions proposed in the book and, thirdly suggest three interrelated concepts aimed at informing and extending our understanding of interprofessional simulation. The final section, in turn, will suggest some directions for further research on simulation-based interprofessional learning implied by the turn to practice.

H. Rystedt (✉)
University of Gothenburg, Gothenburg, Sweden
e-mail: hans.rystedt@ped.gu.se

M. Abrandt Dahlgren · S. Nyström
Linköping University, Linköping, Sweden
e-mail: madeleine.abrandt.dahlgren@liu.se; sofia.nystrom@liu.se

L. Felländer-Tsai
Karolinska Institutet, Stockholm, Sweden
e-mail: li.tsai@ki.se

© Springer Nature Switzerland AG 2019
M. Abrandt Dahlgren et al. (eds.), *Interprofessional Simulation in Health Care*,
Professional and Practice-based Learning 26,
https://doi.org/10.1007/978-3-030-19542-7_9

9.2   Empirical Contributions to Simulation Pedagogy

A central principle in designing for learning is the quest for coherence between the intended learning outcomes, design, teaching and assessment, which has been addressed in terms of *constructive alignment* (e.g. Biggs 1996; Biggs and Tang 2011). However, on the basis of the empirical chapters in Part II we would suggest that the meaning of constructive alignment could be broadened to account for the open-ended nature of simulation activities. As instantiated in a series of chapters in this book, simulations, that at a first glance might be seen as similar, may imply different understandings among learners (Sect. 5.2). Further, it is argued that the learners' understanding of a scenario is highly dependent on how it is framed in briefings (Sect. 4.2); through in-scenario instructions (Sect. 4.3); and the location of the activities (Sects. 5.2 and 6.2). The conclusion that simulations unfold differently in various contexts imply that the outcomes are more or less open-ended. For this reason, it might be hard to state in advance, at least on a detailed level, how the outcomes should be defined and assessed. This however, does not mean that the outcomes of certain designs are random and that the concept of constructive alignment should be abandoned. Rather the results of the chapters in the book point to needs for extending the notion of constructive alignment to account for the emergent and local contingencies of simulation activities. Such a reformulation, we believe, point to the possibility to account for how different material arrangements, technological set-ups, localities, instructions etc. could be aligned to promote interprofessional learning. So, in sum, we would stress that the consistency between outcomes, design, teaching and assessment should be extended to considerations on how these elements and their relations are formed in moment-to-moment interactions and the set-up of the learning environment. On this basis, we will turn to how various ways of *preparing for simulations*, *doing interprofessional simulation* and *arranging for reflection* may provide different opportunities for what is possible to learn.

9.2.1   Preparing for Interprofessional Simulation

A question, of particular concern in this book, is how to design simulation activities to ensure a focus on critical aspects of efficient interprofessional teamwork. How to prepare participants and plan for learning is thus crucial, both from the participants' and facilitators' perspective. In prior research, much attention has been paid to how to design simulation-environments in ways that represent important aspects of the work environment and the tasks to be trained. It is widely acknowledged that there are always differences between simulations and "real-world" tasks that have to be accounted for. One way, to address this gap is to prepare the participants for the specific conditions of the simulation and how actions should be carried out in comparison to clinical work. Drawing on familiarity with work, however, raises questions on how to prepare novice learners for tasks they lack work experiences of (see Sect. 4.2). An additional question, addressed in Sect. 4.3, is how to design for in-scenario instructions to compensate for simulators' lack of displaying the variety of cues available in face-to-face encounters with patients in clinical settings.

When it comes to insufficient knowledge among novice students of the task to be performed, Sect. 4.2 shows how instructions in the simulator environment could be utilized as a means by facilitators to demonstrate and assess students' knowledge, both on the performance of technical procedures and applying teamwork principles. Further, the chapter shows how formative assessments of the students displayed understandings provide necessary means for corrections and re-demonstrations of importance for the upcoming scenario. Since scenarios involving both performance of technical procedures and how to collaborate in teams such scenarios might be too complex and overwhelming for novice learners. This matter seems especially important since such scenarios entangle the coordination of multiple skills, roles and perspectives needed for concerted teamwork. Therefore, we would argue that preparing students through discrete instructions step-by-step could be helpful for novice learners to gain from simulations in general and interprofessional simulations in particular.

In the training of interprofessional teamwork it seems utterly important how to compensate for the "chronic insufficiency" of simulators (Chap. 4) to display the variety of signs and cues available in encounters with human beings. For facilitators, this implies considerations on to what extent the simulator displays the necessary information and, as addressed in this chapter, how much additional information the participants need before entering simulations and/or during scenarios. Surprisingly few studies have addressed the need for in-scenario instructions (brought up in Sect. 4.3) in order for participants to understand what disorders the simulator is intended to represent and to respond accordingly. Further, as shown in Sect. 4.3, the forms of such instructions need to be aligned to the intended learning outcomes, since different forms of in-scenario instructions could be more suited to novices (learning step-by-step) whilst others fulfil goals of keeping the momentum in scenarios of acute situations taylored for professional teams (see also Escher et al. 2017).

In designing for interprofessional simulation it is crucial to focus on the most critical features of team collaboration to be successful. As presented in Sect. 4.3, CRM principles could serve as a tool for achieving this, as for instance how to make efficient use of each other's competencies in joint problem-solving by highlighting each other's roles and responsibilities. Further, Sect. 4.3 points to needs for an all-embracing model that ensure constructive alignment (Biggs 1996). Another important contribution is the need to carefully consider the complexity of scenarios with respect to the objectives of training interprofessional collaboration, for instance by downplaying the difficulty of technical skills to promote an attention to team collaboration and interprofessional issues.

9.2.2 Doing Interprofessional Simulation

An attunement to each other's action is identified as a crucial feature of concerted teamwork (Hindmarsh and Pilnick 2002) and connects to central principles of Crew Resource Management (CRM), such as to coordinate and to support other team members (Miller et al. 2014). By introducing the notions of *in and out of synchrony* Sect. 5.3 provides new insights in how the needs for coordination and shared understandings could be made visible in interprofessional simulations. In line with Hindmarsh and Pilnick (2002), the chapter brings attention to the fluidity and the visibility of bodily positions and actions characterizing coordinated teamwork. Thereby, the notions provide conceptual tools to design scenarios for promoting interprofessional collaboration and to evaluate in what ways the design supports interactions that meet the intended objectives of the scenario. Several of the chapters in this book align to the rationale for training together to be able to work together and deal with how different *locations* offer different opportunities for learning and how the observers' possibilities for deliberate noticing could be enhanced. Bringing attention to the observers' possibilities for learning and the differences between spaces are substantial since most simulations presuppose that all learners are not given opportunities to take part in scenarios and that all, or a large part of training, is assigned to observing.

Especially, Sect. 5.2 provide important insights in how the conditions for participants to develop their medical, affective and communicative knowledge varies between different locations, i.e. inside the simulation, operator and reflection room, respectively. Whilst participating in the scenario provides opportunities to draw on, enact and extend their medical knowledge it also involves affective and communicative dimensions. For students, taking an observers' role together with an instructor in the operator room, the conditions for learning are radically different. Here, instructors can direct the participants' attention to critical aspects of teamwork and elaborate on medical and communicative aspects in form of occasioned mini-lectures. Affective dimensions, however, are more backgrounded in the operator room but arise anew in the reflection room where all participants meet face to face. Both participants acting in the scenario and observers are asked to bring up their views on what happened, which opens for reflections on all knowledge dimensions in a collegial interprofessional manner. An important take-home message is that different locations both enable and de-limit the possibilities for learning and reflection and, most important, that affordances of the different locations are essential to consider in designing simulation.

The conclusion that location is critical for the possibilities to learn is also brought up in Sect. 6.2, but in this case with a focus on *proximate observation* (from the operator room) in comparison to *distant observations* (through a video link). A major conclusion is that the former encourages engagement and possibilities for active observations, whilst the latter is characterized as passive with limited possibilities for novices to discern events of significance for interprofessional teamwork. This passivity, it is argued, could be compensated by means of observation scripts, but as mentioned in the commentary by O'Keeffe such scripts might not fully compensate for this matter. Further, O'Keeffe suggests that the differences between proximate and distant observations might to a larger extent be a result of the instructors' guidance (in the operator room), or lack thereof (in distant observations), than the location per se.

In line with the previous chapter, the following one addresses the possibilities for extending the outcomes for observers through scripts (Sect. 6.3). Drawing on Tanner's (2006) concept of *noticing* as core component of clinical judgement in nursing the authors present how students observing simulations could be prompted to evaluate the performance of their peers in scenarios. A revision of observer guides in line with Tanner's and empirical findings showed that the logic of the students' comments shifted from superficial evaluations to noticing. This shift implied that the students were guided to "read" the unfolding context, identify significant features and make predictions on what should be done next. Further, the authors suggest that such guides could be beneficial for enhancing students' generic capacities for noticing and judgment in clinical practice. Whether or not this conclusion holds, the chapter provides an excellent example of how a theoretical framework could be applied to make a substantial and practical contribution to how observers attention could be directed to significant features of scenarios. Although the empirical example concerns uni-professional teamwork, the chapter could also inform how to design simulation training to ensure that the participants' attention is directed to interprofessional facets of collaboration. But, as the authors argue, the focus of attention cannot be achieved solely by observer protocols, but also need to be prepared for in briefings or pre-briefings and, as addressed in next section, through deliberate reflection.

9.2.3 Arranging for Reflection

Feedback has been identified to be the most important condition for learners to benefit from simulations (Issenberg et al. 2005). Further, the notion of reflection and how it is intertwined with learning has been a central topic for theorisation of learning for decades (Schön 1983). It has also been picked up as a central concept to understand learning processes in post-simulation briefings (e.g. Fanning and Gaba 2007; Rudolph et al. 2006; Eikeland Husebø et al. 2015). Still, there are a vast range of questions that could be further explored by digging deeper in what actually takes place in debriefings.

A principal question, addressed in Sect. 7.2, is how different debriefing models enter in the participants' discussions and in what ways they are consequential for what is thematised. Drawing on video data on the training of interprofessional student teams at two Swedish simulation centres, the chapter explores different practical understandings of debriefing and their consequences. It is argued that one of them, *debriefing as algorithm*, pre-figure a step-by-step procedure in which examples of good professional practice were emphasised as a basis for the lessons to be learned. Such an understanding also implied that spontaneous reflections from the students were less likely to be brought up as topics for discussion. Another understanding, debriefing as *laissez-faire*, implied an informal format in which participants were asked to bring up whatever came to their mind. This gave more room for the students' individual learning needs in comparison to the understanding of debriefing as algorithm. However, as claimed in Sect. 7.2, neither of these understandings could guarantee an attention to interprofessional issues, since discussions on inter-professional learning as such were mainly absent in both cases and medical topics tended to overshadow issues on collaboration. In comparison to the student teams, an analysis of debriefing of professionals showed that many of the features are shared, but also that there are important differences. The authors point out that the ways of emphasising "chains of action", characterising the debriefing of professionals, highlights the interdependence between the participants' actions that could further their understanding of teamwork, something that could also be highly beneficial for debriefing students.

Section 7.3 has another take on debriefings by focusing on the interplay between questions and responses for shaping the students' understandings of video-clips from scenarios just performed. Whilst the previous Sect. (7.2) concludes that neither of the models under study could assure an interprofessional focus, this chapter offer a model for considering the use of open-ended versus specific introductions to video-clips. Further, it is claimed in Sect. 7.3 that students' understanding of video recorded scenarios is not only a result of the video itself, but rather how it is introduced and the discussions that follow. In addition to Sect. 7.2, suggesting that debriefings should aim for recontextualizations of scenarios, the analysis in Sect. 7.3 illustrates how students' initial formulations can be re-formulated and re-conceptualised through the facilitators' questions and peer-student contributions. Another conclusion is that the students orient to various facets of collaboration of central concern for interprofessional teamwork. Although they do not address such issues on a meta-level, their discussions are evidently directed to their professional conduct and how they act together as a team.

To sum up the chapter on debriefing, it can be concluded that debriefing models can influence the forms of interaction and the issues that will be thematised. In Sect. 7.2 it is formulated as different practical understandings pre-determine how debriefings will be played out. This, however, should not be understood in a deterministic way, that the outcomes of a model are given in advance. Rather, as argued in the theoretical part in this book (Chap. 2), the outcomes of how simulation activities are designed could be more or less likely, but still are open-ended. However, why and how simulation activities can take different directions is developed further in Sect. 7.3 by showing how debriefings will unfold is a result of moment-to-moment interactions between facilitators and participants in which the focus of attention can be changed in every next turn. So, what are the lessons to be learned? We would argue that the choice of debriefing model matters, but no model itself guarantee a focus on interprofessional issues. Rather, we would suggest that the pedagogical development of debriefing practices should pay careful attention to how to promote reflections on an interactional level, for instance how different formulations of facilitators' questions and prompts are critical for whether interprofessional issues will be thematised or not. Further, we believe that such considerations could be a way to direct the participants' attention to "chains of actions" (7.2), i.e. how actions, consequences, roles and responsibilities are intertwined and hang together as a critical condition for interprofessional teamwork.

9.3 Methodological Contributions

The insights in interprofessional simulation practices presented in this chapter are enabled by theories and methodological tools that give prominence to the practice itself and collaborative aspects of learning. The theoretical and methodological tools (Chaps. 2 and 3) rely on a solid base of theoretical assumptions. The *Practice theory* approach takes its point of departure in a conceptualization of how our social and material world is constituted which give prominence to emergent character of how simulations are enacted. The approach conducted under the umbrella of *Situated action* in this book share this assumption on a general level, but instead of theory as a starting point for the analysis, the analytical focus is directed to the members' own methods for achieving a shared understanding of situations. Consequently, there are both differences and similarities between approaches and what knowledge on interprofessional learning that they can contribute with.

First, the different approaches provide different kinds of results. Whilst both studies based on theories of situated action and practice theory share an interest for how social order is constituted, analyses carried out from a practice theory perspective are guided by the core concepts of the theory and the empirical findings are to a large extent framed in theoretical terms. In comparison, analyses under the umbrella of situated action end up with detailed accounts of a significant array of the participants' own methods for achieving shared understandings and concerted actions (for a further discussion see Chap. 2 this volume).

Secondly, both approaches emphasize collaborative analyses as prominent, but the analyses are carried out on different levels of detail (see Sects. 3.2 and 3.3). In the studies based on practice theory, video data are subjected to the identification of significant activities through observations and comparative analyses, whilst the unit of analysis in EM/CA informed studies of situated action consists of talk-in-interaction and how shared understandings are built up sequentially. For instance, analyses relying on practice theory and related socio-material approaches point out how simulation activities involve different locations with different opportunities for learning (Sect. 5.2); how various understandings of the simulator as a body are related to different knowledge domains and possibilities for knowledge development (Sect. 5.3) and how different arrangement for observations are highly influential for students' attention, engagement and reflection (Sects. 6.2 and 6.3). In comparison, studies on situated action could demonstrate how the students' conduct unfold in cycles of activities involving demonstrations, assessments and re-demonstrations (Sect. 4.2); through timely/occasioned in-scenario instructions (Sect. 4.3) and the significance of facilitators' questions and peer-contributions for shaping the students' understanding of video-recorded scenarios (Sect. 7.3).

Thirdly, the results carried out under the umbrella of the two approaches may appear as somewhat divergent when it comes to interprofessional learning. On the one hand, the chapters relying on a practice theory framework claim that interprofessional issues are treated as more or less peripheral by the participants in the empirical settings (e.g. Sects. 6.2 and 7.2). On the other hand, the studies of situated action, claim that the participants orient to many of the core principles involved in coordinating teamwork, for instance when taking positions in a team (Sect. 4.2) and reflecting on how to communicate and collaborate effectively with each other in an interprofessional team (Sect. 7.3). This matter may be due to the differences in analytical commitments. Whilst the analyses informed by practice theory take the thematisation of interprofessional learning on a conceptual level as a point of departure, studies on situated action try to un-pack the members' methods and the resources they employ to make sense of each other's actions in the situation at hand (see Sect. 2.2). However, each contribution is relevant for understanding interprofessional learning since both a conceptualisation of interprofessional collaboration on a meta-level and reflecting on teamwork on a concrete level can be regarded as relevant forms of reflection-on-action that are critical for participants to learn from simulations (see also Schön 1983; Eikeland Husebø et al. 2015; Rudolph et al. 2006).

9.4   Conceptual Contributions

In addition to the empirical and methodological contributions summarized above, the ambition is also to contribute with a conceptual development that can aid future research. We would suggest *three interrelated concepts* to be at core of what the turn to practice and our chapters imply for understanding interprofessional learning in and through simulations. These concepts refer to three aspects that are regarded as constituting each other, pointing to that it is the relation between them that is of primary concern. The first one is *materiality*, implying a focus on the material properties of simulations and how various locations and arrangements play a significant role in shaping opportunities for interprofessional learning. The second concept, *embodiment*, draws attention to how simulators are designed to approach a human patient and how manikins can be reconstituted in multiple ways in their use. Further, the concept refers to embodied aspects of professional knowledge and conduct. The third concept, *interaction*, puts the focus on how facilitators and learners are able to achieve shared understandings of simulated events in and through interaction in the technological environment (see Fig. 9.1).

Fig. 9.1 Three interrelated core concepts highlighting how the understanding of learning in interprofessional simulations is bound together with the material, embodied and interactional aspects and the interdependence between them

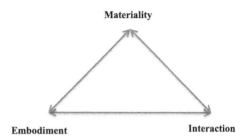

Materiality

Embodiment   Interaction

9.4.1 *Materiality*

A shared point of departure following the Turn to practice, is that our understanding of learning in simulations presupposes analyses of how activities are intertwined with artefacts, objects and other material properties of the environment (see Sect. 2). This stance put the analytical focus on how material entities are entangled with processes in which participants in simulations create a share meaning of the activities they are engaged in. Throughout the chapters, there is a vast range of instances of how material objects matter. As demonstrated in Sect. 4.2, in the case of briefings, the chain of demonstrations, assessments and re-demonstrations are all intrinsically intertwined with the manikin and the physical space. Following such sequences of interactions, provide instances of the *material grounds* for learning in which the instructions have visible consequences for the novice students' increased mastery of technical procedures and how to take positions for coordinating the team. The following Sect. (4.3), demonstrates how in-scenario instructions could radically transform the ways in which the simulation is understood. This means that simulators are material objects that are *flexibly interpretable* by being highly dependent on how they are shaped in and through interaction. This openness however, could be problematic when simulators are to be used to address specific learning goals. For this reason, we would emphasize that the ways in which activities are designed to compensate for the simulators shortcomings is absolutely decisive for what is possible to learn (Sect. 4.3). In line with Escher et al. (2017), we would suggest that the methods for in-scenario instructions really matter. In short, this means that one cannot understand the impact of the material properties of simulations without accounting for the practices through which they are brought to life.

Another instance of the significance of materiality is provided by Sects. 5.2 and 6.2, showing that the *location* of activities provides entirely different affordances for instruction, learning and reflection. Similarly, as attended in Sect. 7.3, *video* provides shared visual grounds for not only re-actualizing what took place in the scenario, but also to re-formulate and re-conceptualize what was just shown into professional and interprofessional concerns. Extending the notion of materiality, the *debriefing models* could also be seen as instances of objects of decisive importance for how discussions are played out. For instance, facilitators' questions on "what went well?" (Sect. 7.3) draws on a model with a physical counterpart on posters in the debriefing rooms, prompting the participants to respond accordingly and being corrected when they do not deliver a preferred answer. Similarly, *observation guides*, could be decisive for directing the participants' focus to be in line with the intended learning objectives and with possibilities to contribute to participants' development of generic capacities for noticing (Sect. 6.3).

In all, these examples contribute to the ever-lasting discussion on fidelity, suspension of disbelief and its implications for learning. At large, the view of fidelity as to merely concern a superficial similarity between the simulation and what is simulated has been rejected. Instead, issues on fidelity have been reformulated to concern to what extent the simulation approaches the learning objectives of the training (Hamstra et al. 2014; Schoenherr and Hamstra 2017; Tun et al. 2015). We agree with this position but would add that it is not the material properties of simulations, nor the pedagogical design per se that are decisive for what is possible to learn from interprofessional simulations. Instead, we suggest that the interpretation flexibility of technologies points to the interplay between these entities as paving the way for learning. As pointed out by Rooney et al. (2015, p. 276), fidelity could be seen as "…an emergent phenomenon that must be constantly worked at, socially and materially, in order to be produced and maintained". What is meant, can be illustrated by the way facilitators provide in-scenario instructions, taking both the material features of the simulator and the participants' actions as basis for adding what is needed for them to understand what the simulation is a simulation of (Escher et al. 2017; Hopwood et al. 2016).

The perspective on fidelity, as proposed above, points to a need for revisiting the notion of transfer. Instead of attending to physical or psychological similarities between the simulation and the workplace, we would suggest an approach to simulations as practices in their own right. Such a focus put the analytical focus on how participants in interprofessional simulations relate to such similarities themselves. By asking "What is being simulated" (Hopwood et al. 2016, p. 170) it is possible answer questions on in what ways simulation activities are relevant for the tasks to be trained and the intended learning objectives. As illustrated in many of the chapters in the book it can offer insights in what kind of issues that are thematised, for instance in what ways they are relevant for foregrounding critical aspects of collaboration. Answering this question can also exemplify the material grounds (simulators, spaces, guides, models, video etc.) to direct a shared attention among participants to critical facets of interprofessional teamwork.

9.4.2 Embodiment

The notion of embodiment takes different, but complementary, meanings throughout the chapters. Firstly, the notion brings attention to the embodied character of professional *knowledge* involved in concerted interprofessional teamwork. Secondly, the notion denotes how human features are represented in the process of *designing* simulators. Thirdly, it refers to how simulators are *used* in interprofessional training and how simulators could convey multiple understandings of the body.

Starting with the embodied character of *professional knowledge*, we stated in Chap. 2 that, interprofessional teamwork relies on "the tacit order" in which the sequential organisation of non-verbal actions, such as gestures and use of equipment, provide visible and recognisable means for team members to understand and coordinate procedures, for instance when anaesthetising patients (Hindmarsh and Pilnick 2002). A critical question, thus, is how simulations can contribute to educate learners with various levels of expertise to develop such competencies. In line with the theoretical reasons for turning to practice, we would argue that much knowledge involved in teamwork, that might at a first glance be regarded as tacit, is possible to explicate and train through simulations. For instance, as shown in Sect. 4.2, the task to take the leaders position in resuscitation teamwork can be, not only, demonstrated and explained by means of the simulation environment, but also how simulations can provide tools for assessing the students' *displayed* understanding of the leaders' responsibilities for coordinating teamwork. Further, the same chapter points to the needs for going beyond assessments of students' claimed understandings and how simulations provide resources for demonstrating and assessing the participants' embodied knowledge. Further, simulations provide opportunities for facilitators to make use of the participants' performance during scenarios to direct observers' attention to critical actions, positionings, roles and responsibilities, as for instance team-coordination when turning a "vomiting patient" (Sect. 6.2). In a similar vein, video provides resources for facilitators, and learners alike, to re-actualise embodied aspect of what took place in preceding scenarios, such as what it means to act in a calm and respectful manner in front of patients (Sect. 7.3).

As pointed out in Chap. 8, the process of *designing* simulators does not involve a mere replication of the human body, but first and foremost involves the features of the body that are relevant for the activity in which it will be used. This point is exemplified by the way in which body fat could be represented in gynaecological simulators, illustrating that it is not the physical properties of fat per se that are desirable. Rather it is the feeling when examining internal organs through specific procedures, which in turn, shows how the design of the simulated body is bound up with particular examination practices.

Further, Chap. 8, draws attention to the embodiment of simulators in their *use* by distinguishing between three modes of thinking about simulators' reality. First, the physical mode of thinking in quantitative terms, secondly the semantical mode of thinking, understandings tied to particular communities of practice, and thirdly the phenomenal mode of thinking, foregrounding the user experiences. However, as demonstrated in Sect. 5.3, the users may relate to the simulator in different ways as the scenario unfolds: as a technical, medical and human body, respectively. Still, the modes of thinking suggested above could be highly relevant, since the ways in which students engaged with the manikin and the tasks they performed, "reflected some of their specific professional roles and responsibilities but were also enacted as incentives to initiate or coordinate collaborative efforts" (Chap. 8). As suggested in Chap. 8, different ways of constructing the body in the intersection between its purpose and its users can provide some insights in how simulators can be designed and used in the context of interprofessional learning, "The different practices of healthcare in the different disciplines and professions practice the body, feel the body, interact with the body in different ways" (Chap. 8). The understanding of these differences can inform the design of simulators that render domain specific knowledge visible and contribute to an awareness of each other's roles and responsibilities as a cornerstone for coordinated teamwork (see also Oxelmark et al. 2017).

In sum, the notion of embodiment, as suggested in this book, involves the interaction between the learners' body and the simulated body, in the sense that simulators need to support essential aspects of professional and interprofessional activities, including tasks, roles and responsibilities. But as pointed out in Sect. 5.3, the enactment of the body during simulations is fluid and can take different form throughout the simulation and offer various opportunities for learning. This in turn, points to how the meaning of simulators and simulations alike is intrinsically bound up with how interactions between learners unfolds in relation to the local contingencies and the material environment, a conclusion that will be further elaborated in the section on interaction that follows.

9.4.3   Interaction

The notion of interaction is of twofold interest in throughout the book. First, it serves as an *analytical tool* for performing in-depth investigations of how participants in a simulation environment engage with it each other and the material environment to understand and respond to the unfolding events. Secondly, the interest in interaction is premised on the assumption that *learning together* is of critical importance for developing capacities at the core of interprofessional teamwork. Thereby, it is of critical concern how we can design for interactions that highlight interprofessional issues.

As noted in previous sections on Materiality and Embodiment, and the qualities these concepts embrace, are not to be regarded as sufficient for understanding the conditions for learning themselves. Although an understanding of how material and embodied features enter in and provide essential prerequisites for learning, learning in interprofessional simulations can only be fully grasped by and understanding of how these aspects come together and are brought to bear in and through interaction. This points on the one hand, to the concept of Interaction as an intrinsic precondition for learning and, on the other, to the interrelatedness of Materiality, Embodiment and Interaction. The critical question from this point of view is how to design for interaction, not only between facilitators, observers and participants acting in the scenario, but also how to pave the way for relevant interactions with the simulator and other material properties of the learning environment.

Many of the means for enabling and promoting interaction has already been touched upon. Sect. 4.2 points to how *explicit instructions* are essential in demonstrating for novice students how to perform manual procedures and how to coordinate teamwork. This also demonstrates how various forms of formative assessments function as a basis for instructions. In this way, incorrect performance, as displayed by students in the simulation environment, is deliberately acted upon by facilitators to adjust and re-demonstrate how tasks should be formed to be in accordance with established guidelines. Similarly, as noted in Sect. 4.3, the participants' actions in relation to the simulator form the preconditions necessary for providing *in-scenario instructions* that are sensitive to the participants' understanding the scenario to direct them to proceed in alignment with the intended learning objectives. Another way of directing the participants' attention and activities is through *observer guidelines* as suggested in Sect. 6.2 and further developed in Sect. 6.3. In doing this, these chapters also show how to enable an active role of observers, not only for the sake of their own learning, but also for the possibilities to make use of these observations in debriefings to bring up relevant themes and to support focused discussion. Most importantly, providing these forms of instructions, could contribute to direct learners' attention to interprofessional issues. Thereby, such instruction could provide solutions to a problem raised in some of the chapters, that medical issues tend to overshadow the thematization of collaborative concerns.

Still another form of instructions to promote interaction and reflection is to make deliberate use of *pedagogical models*. As shown in Sects. 7.2 and 7.3, the practical understandings of debriefing, partly conveyed by articulated models, are consequential for both the content and structure of the discussions. In this way, the choice of pedagogical model can enable and delimit both what can be brought up as a topic for discussion and the participants' possibilities to contribute. But, as pointed out in Sect. 7.3, the direction of debriefing discussions is open-ended in the sense that it can take new directions in every next turn. As a consequence, it is necessary to account for how the facilitators' instruction in form of initiations and questions can promote reflections and contribute to transform the participants' understanding of their own performance and its relevance for interprofessional collaboration (Sect. 7.3).

A final remark on instruction, and of specific concern for debriefings, is the possibilities to draw on what took place in the scenario as a basis for reflection and generalisation to interprofessional contexts beyond the immediate situation. An established method for re-actualizing what happened is to start debriefings with questions on what happened and ask participants to recapitulate how they experienced the situation (e.g. Steinwachs 1992). Although, making such rounds might be important and purposeful to establish a shared view as a basis for further analysis, it has also been criticised for overshadowing opportunities for deepened reflections (Kihlgren et al. 2015). Drawing on the chapters in this book, we would point to the significance of material objects as a means for instructions to promote focused reflections. As mentioned above, different forms of observer scripts and guidelines could serve these goals, but also different forms of visualising critical moments of scenarios or their development over time. As shown in Sect. 7.3, video recordings provide an exemplary tool, but we would also open up for other forms for visualisation that enable instructors to encourage reconsiderations on what took place in another light. Hopefully, such experiences could contribute to extend the lessons learned in simulation contexts to interprofessional collaboration at work.

To conclude, the turn to practice implies that interaction stands out as a core concepts both for understanding and arranging for interprofessional learning. However, as depicted in Fig. 9.1, none of the concepts can account for understanding simulation activity in its entirety. Instead, we would suggest that the relations between them could be a useful starting point, since we believe that a consideration of their interdependence can contribute to a more comprehensive understanding of learning in and through interprofessional simulation practice.

9.5   Future Research

An all over argument of the research presented in this book is that we need to open up "the black box" of interprofessional simulation practice to understand the conditions for learning, but also to inform educational practices and future research. In following the idiom that "the devil is in the detail" we would emphasise how simulations activities unfold as a result of the participants' understanding of the situation as displayed through their concrete actions. From this follows that future research would benefit from studies that pay close attention to how the directions of briefings, scenarios and debriefings are highly sensitive to how facilitators formulate questions, prompts and so on, but also how the simulation training is framed in a wider sense. Whilst pedagogical models might be supportive for designing, executing and evaluating simulation activities, the series of studies presented in this book, demonstrate that models do not determine the actions to follow. Instead every model needs to be instantiated in concrete actions under the specific circumstances at hand, something that is highly dependent on the facilitators' guidance, instruction and sensitivity for the participants' responses (see also Suchman 1987). From this point of view, we believe that the simulation society would benefit from more research that account for the local and practical contingencies involved in simulation training. Further, we believe that the outcomes of such a research agenda could not only provide a basis for designing interprofessional team training tailored to learners with different backgrounds, but also to inform education for instructors. Although such education necessarily includes models and guidelines as resources for future instructors to learn the tricks of the trade, we think that an increased emphasis on how simulations unfold in the course of action could be a valuable contribution to develop pedagogical strategies that are sensitive to the intricate details of learning in and through interprofessional simulations.

References

Biggs, J. (1996). Enhancing teaching through constructive alignment. *The International Journal of Higher Education Research, 32*, 347. https://doi.org/10.1007/BF00138871.

Biggs, J., & Tang, C. S. (2011). *Teaching for quality learning at university: What the student does.* Maidenhead: McGraw-Hill. ISBN: 9780335242757.

Eikeland Husebø, S., O'Regan, S., & Nestel, D. (2015). Reflective practice and its role in simulation. *Clinical Simulation in Nursing, 11*(8), 368–375. https://doi.org/10.1016/j.ecns.2015.04.005.

Escher, C., Rystedt, H., Creutzfeldt, J., Meurling, L., Nyström, S., Dahlberg, J., et al. (2017). Method matters: Impact of in-scenario instruction on simulation-based team training. *Advances in Simulation, 2*, 25. https://doi.org/10.1186/s41077-017-0059-9.

Fanning, R. M., & Gaba, D. M. (2007). The role of debriefing in simulation-based learning. *Simulation in Healthcare, 2*(2), 115–125.

Hamstra, S. J., Brydges, R., Hatala, R., Zendejas, B., & Cook, D. A. (2014). Reconsidering fidelity in simulation-based training. *Academic Medicine, 89*(3), 387–392. https://doi.org/10.1097/ACM.0000000000000130.

Hindmarsh, J., & Pilnick, A. (2002). The tacit order of teamwork: Collaboration and embodied conduct in anesthesia. *The Sociological Quarterly, 43*(2), 139–164. https://doi.org/10.1111/j.1533-8525.2002.tb00044.x.

Hopwood, N., Rooney, D., Boud, D., & Kelly, M. (2016). Simulation in higher education: A socio-material view. *Educational Philosophy and Theory, 48*(2), 167–178. https://doi.org/10.1080/00131857.2014.971403.

Issenberg, B. S., McGaghie, W. C., Petrusa, E. R., Lee, G. D., & Scalese, R. J. (2005). Features and uses of high-fidelity medical simulations that leads to effective learning: A BEME systematic review. *Medical Teacher, 27*(1), 10–28.

Kihlgren, P., Spanager, L., & Dieckmann, P. (2015). Investigating novice doctors' reflections in debriefings after simulation scenarios. *Medical Teacher, 37*(5), 437–443. https://doi.org/10.3109/0142159X.2014.956054.

Miller, R. D., Eriksson, L. I., Fleisher, L. A., Wiener-Kronish, J. P., Cohen, N. H., & Young, W. L. (2014). *Miller's anesthesia E-Book.* Amsterdam: Elsevier Health Sciences.

Oxelmark, L., Nordahl Amorøe, T., Carlzon, L., & Rystedt, H. (2017). Students' understanding of teamwork and professional roles after interprofessional simulation—A qualitative analysis. *Advances in Simulation, 2*, 8. https://doi.org/10.1186/s41077-017-0041-6.

Rooney, D., Hopwood, N., Boud, D., & Kelly, M. (2015). The role of simulation in pedagogies of higher education for the health professions: Through a practice-based lens. *Vocations and Learning, 8*(3), 269–285. https://doi.org/10.1007/s12186-015-9138-z.

Rudolph, J. W., Simon, R., Dufresne, R. L., & Raemer, D. B. (2006). There's no such thing as «nonjudgmental» debriefing: A theory and method for debriefing with good judgment. *Simulation in Healthcare, 1*(1), 49–55.

Schoenherr, J. R., & Hamstra, S. J. (2017). Beyond fidelity: Deconstructing the seductive simplicity of fidelity in simulator-based education in the health care professions. *Simulation in Healthcare, 12*(2), 117–123. https://doi.org/10.1097/sih.0000000000000226.

Schön, D. (1983). *The reflective practitioner.* New York: Basic Books.

Steinwachs, B. (1992). How to facilitate a debriefing. *Simulation & Gaming, 23*(2), 186–195. https://doi.org/10.1177/1046878192232006.

Suchman, L. (1987). *Plans and situated actions: The problem of human-machine communication.* Cambridge: Cambridge University Press. ISBN-13: 978–0521331371.

Tanner, C. (2006). Thinking like a nurse: A researched-based model of clinical judgment in nursing. *Journal of Nursing Education, 45*(6), 204–211.

Tun, J. K., Alinier, G., Tang, J., & Kneebone, R. L. (2015). Redefining simulation fidelity for healthcare education. *Simulation & Gaming, 46*(2), 159–174. https://doi.org/10.1177/1046878115576103.

CPSIA information can be obtained
at www.ICGtesting.com
Printed in the USA
LVHW082354090919
630540LV00007B/137/P

9 783030 195410